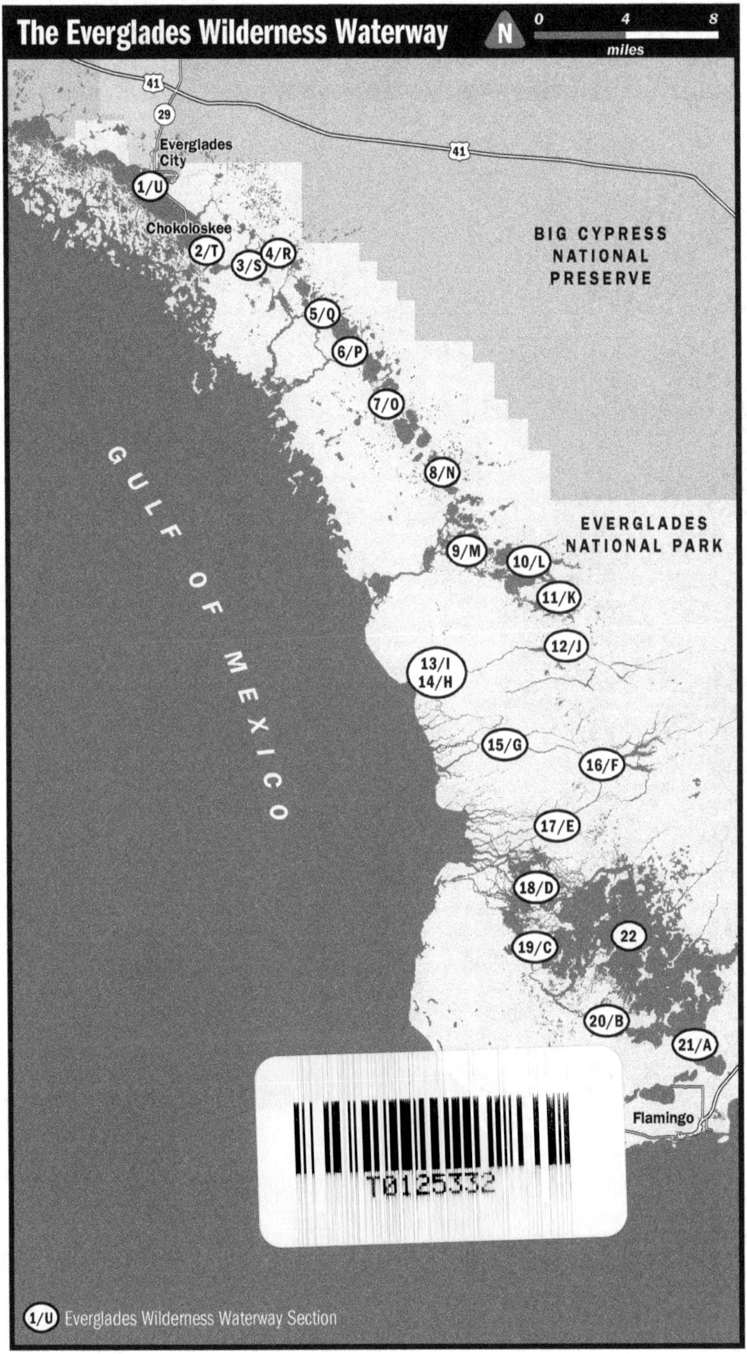
The Everglades Wilderness Waterway
N
0
4
8
miles
41
29
Everglades City
1/U
Chokoloskee
2/T
3/S
4/R
BIG CYPRESS NATIONAL PRESERVE
5/Q
6/P
7/O
8/N
GULF OF MEXICO
EVERGLADES NATIONAL PARK
9/M
10/L
11/K
12/J
13/I
14/H
15/G
16/F
17/E
18/D
22
19/C
20/B
21/A
Flamingo
1/U Everglades Wilderness Waterway Section

The Everglades North & South Day & Overnight Paddles

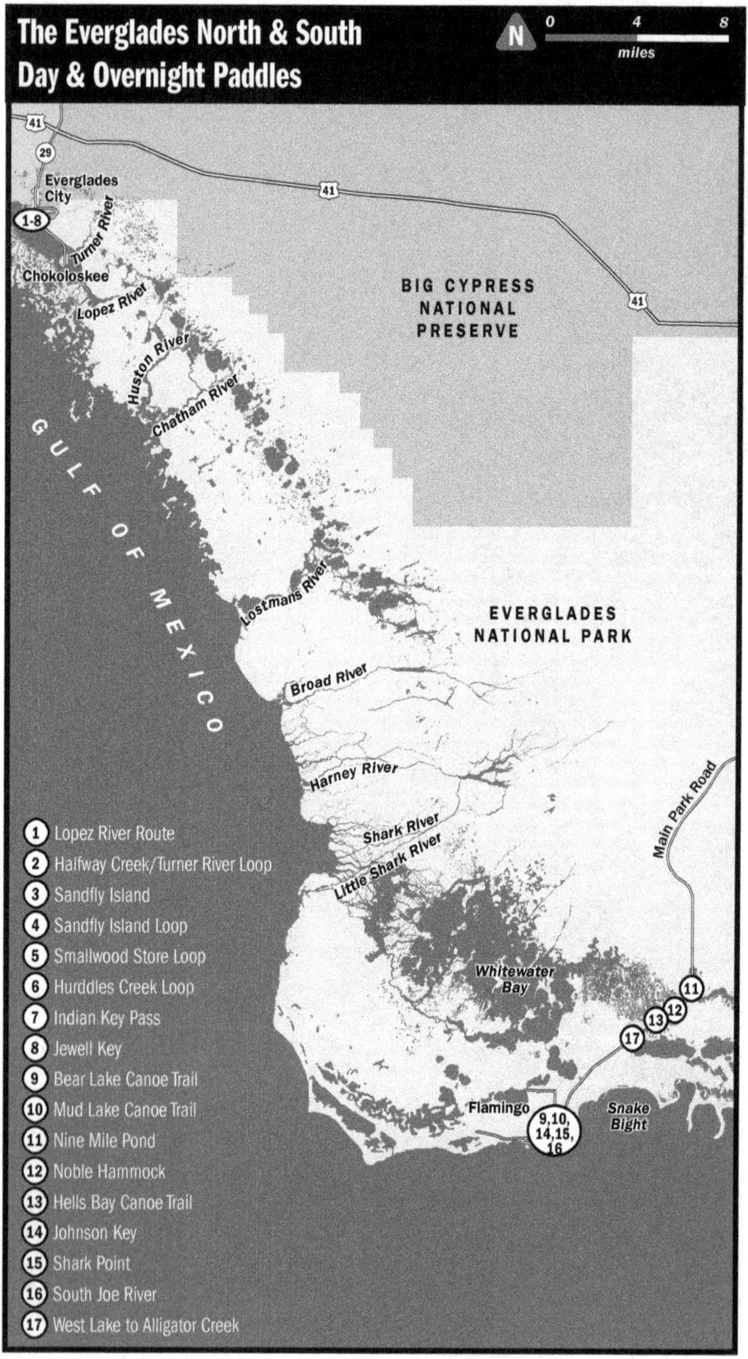
N
0
4
8
miles
41
29
Everglades City
1-8
Turner River
Chokoloskee
Lopez River
Huston River
Chatham River
BIG CYPRESS NATIONAL PRESERVE
GULF OF MEXICO
Lostmans River
EVERGLADES NATIONAL PARK
Broad River
Harney River
Shark River
Little Shark River
Main Park Road
Whitewater Bay
11
12
13
17
Flamingo
9,10, 14,15, 16
Snake Bight
1 Lopez River Route
2 Halfway Creek/Turner River Loop
3 Sandfly Island
4 Sandfly Island Loop
5 Smallwood Store Loop
6 Hurddles Creek Loop
7 Indian Key Pass
8 Jewell Key
9 Bear Lake Canoe Trail
10 Mud Lake Canoe Trail
11 Nine Mile Pond
12 Noble Hammock
13 Hells Bay Canoe Trail
14 Johnson Key
15 Shark Point
16 South Joe River
17 West Lake to Alligator Creek

OVERVIEW MAP KEY

OTHER MENASHA RIDGE PRESS PADDLING GUIDES

The Alaska River Guide

Canoeing & Kayaking Florida

Canoeing & Kayaking Georgia

A Canoeing & Kayaking Guide to Kentucky

A Canoeing & Kayaking Guide to the Ozarks

Canoeing & Kayaking New York

Canoeing & Kayaking West Virginia

Carolina Whitewater

PADDLING THE EVERGLADES WILDERNESS WATERWAY

YOUR ALL-IN-ONE GUIDE TO
FLORIDA'S 99-MILE TREASURE
plus 17 DAY & OVERNIGHT TRIPS

Holly Genzen
Anne McCrary Sullivan

MENASHA RIDGE PRESS
www.menasharidge.com

Paddling the Everglades Wilderness Waterway:
Your All-in-one Guide to Florida's 99-mile Treasure
***plus* 17 Day & Overnight Trips**

Published by Menasha Ridge Press
Printed in the United States of America
Distributed by Publishers Group West
First edition, first printing

Cover design by Scott McGrew
Cartography by Scott McGrew and Holly Genzen
Text design by Annie Long
Cover photographs by Holly Genzen
Authors' photographs by Andrea Hillebrand; photograph on page 13 by Rick Jones
All other interior photographs by Holly Genzen and Anne McCrary Sullivan

Library of Congress Cataloging-in-Publication Data
Genzen, Holly.
Paddling the Everglades wilderness waterway : your all-in-one guide for thru-paddling Florida's 99-mile treasure with additional day trips and overnight paddles / Holly Genzen, Anne McCrary Sullivan.
p. cm.
ISBN-13: 978-0-89732-898-2 (pbk.); ISBN 978-1-63404-228-4 (hardcover)
ISBN-10: 0-89732-898-1
1. Canoes and canoeing—Florida—Everglades National Park—Guidebooks.
2. Everglades National Park (Fla.)—Guidebooks. I. Sullivan, Anne McCrary. II. Title.
GV776.A3-Z.F62E934 2011
797.12209759'39—dc23

2011022231

Menasha Ridge Press
An imprint of AdventureKEEN
2204 First Avenue South, Suite 102
Birmingham, Alabama 35233
menasharidge.com

DISCLAIMER

Paddling the Everglades Wilderness Waterway is meant only as a guide to select paddles in the Everglades. This book does not guarantee paddler safety in any way—you paddle at your own risk. Neither Menasha Ridge Press, Holly Genzen, nor Anne McCrary Sullivan are liable for property loss or damage, personal injury, or death that result in any way from accessing or paddling the waterways described in the following pages. Please read carefully the introduction to this book as well as further safety information from other sources. Familiarize yourself with current weather reports and maps of the area you plan to visit (in addition to the maps provided in this guidebook). Be cognizant of park regulations and always follow them. Do not take chances. Every effort has been made to ensure the accuracy of information throughout this book, and the contents of this publication are believed to be correct at the time of printing. Nevertheless, the publisher cannot accept responsibility for errors or omissions, for changes in details given in this guide, or for the consequences of relying on information provided by the same. Assessments of sites are based on the author's own experience; therefore, descriptions given in this guide necessarily contain an element of subjective opinion, which may not reflect the publisher's opinion or dictate a reader's own experience on another occasion.

Contents

PART FIVE: (continued)

Aerial roots in The Nightmare

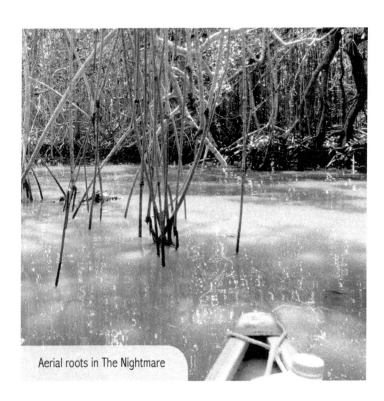

The authors at Picnic Key

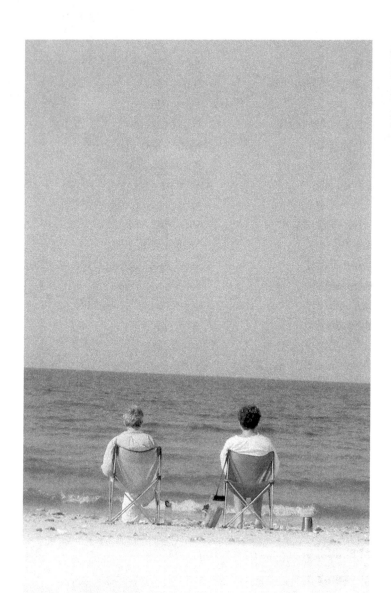

Dedication

For Gary, David, & Jonathan, with love

Holly

**For the family's next generation of paddlers:
Miller, Bremen, Grace, & Anne**

Anne

Acknowledgments

Many people have supported this book, and we are grateful to every one of them. Most notably, we want to thank the personnel of Everglades National Park: Alan Scott, Chief of Interpretation and Visitor Services, whose door was always open to us; Susan Reece, Northwest District Naturalist, and Bob Showler, Flamingo District Interpreter, both of whom tirelessly and with good humor answered our many questions on repeated visits and through e-mails; Mike Jester, Chief of Maintenance; Bill Wagner, Maintenance Supervisor, Northwest District; Rob Neuman, Flamingo Maintenance Supervisor; and a multitude of rangers and volunteers who have provided useful information, especially Shauna Cotrell, and Hampton Hudson, Joe Sterchele, Rita Huston, Tim Taylor, Christi Carmichael, and Dan Blankenship. In the archives of Everglades National Park, Nancy Russell and Bonnie Ciolino helped us dig up whatever elusive details we were seeking.

We are grateful to William G. Truesdell, author of *A Guide to the Wilderness Waterway of the Everglades National Park,* the first guidebook to this maze of mangrove channels. He continues to share with us stories of his days as a naturalist in Everglades National Park and information about the origins of the Waterway.

We have appreciated the assistance of Jon Rizzo, meteorologist at the National Weather Service, Key West, who helped us think through issues of safety related to lightning.

The people of Chokoloskee Island, Everglades City, Florida City, and Flamingo have been welcoming, and operators of marinas, lodges, restaurants, and outfitters have been generous in supplying information about their services and the history of the area. Kenny Brown was especially accommodating; we thank him for sharing his family's long history on Chokoloskee Island and for welcome cups of coffee. Chris Ammerman, postmaster of Chokoloskee, was our smiling informant whenever we had trouble finding people or places. In Everglades City, Bobby Miller provided information and guidance, and Carolyn Thompson at Win-Car Hardware was perennially friendly and helpful.

We've met great people out there in the evenings on the Waterway when we have shared chickees or campsites, and we've heard some entertaining stories. Thanks to all those storytellers! Bill and Mike at Alligator Creek told tales from a long history of thru-paddling the Waterway. Dan and Casey at Johnson Key Chickee, intrepid paddlers out for the first time, without a tent and running out of food, were having the time of their lives and telling a very different story. Nick, who stopped briefly at Plate Creek Chickee, told of odysseys with WaterTribe, a kayaker/canoeist organization, before he headed out again, showing us that paddling in the dark can be a great adventure. A boy on a multiday fishing trip with his father, camping at Willy Willy, grinned and confessed that he was "playing hooky," and on the same evening over dinner on the dock, a kayaker named John shared stories of great places to paddle. Rick, our companion at Harney River Chickee, told of reading many years earlier a newspaper article about thru-paddling the Waterway. He hung on to that clipping and resolved to do the Waterway "someday," and finally, there he was with his boat, *Weeble.* And there was Patrick, traveling with his classic wooden craft, *Old Blue Skies,* who successfully dove under South Joe River Chickee to retrieve a treasured knife, asking us to "watch for sharks."

We also want to thank Manuel, Sven, Anne, and Sandra who came from Germany to thru-paddle the Waterway and who afterward suggested that we tell our readers that one bottle of insect repellent is not enough for four people for 10 days. They made other suggestions that we have incorporated into this book. Deep appreciation goes to Karen and Gary, who gave Holly a ride when she was hitchhiking to Flamingo from the Coot Bay Pond put-in.

Thanks to Jonathan for loaning us *Abigail* on our first thru-paddle and for all the practical support he gave as we worked on this book, and to Margaret, who read every word of the manuscript.

This guidebook would not have been the book it is without the folks at Menasha Ridge Press, particularly our editor, Susan Haynes, who steered this process like a skilled paddler working her way through The Nightmare; Amber Kaye Henderson, who made sure our book was shipshape; and Scott McGrew, who crafted often complex maps with good nature and patience.

Individually, we wish to thank friends and family who offered support and did without when we were tangled in the mangroves or in the manuscript.

Thanks to all my friends who have paddled with me in canoe or kayak.

And deepest appreciation to my family: My parents' inspiration remains with me after all these years—my father, Dr. Herman Kretzschmar, who gave me the wanderlust gene, and my mother, Margaret, who blew the silver whistle when it was time to come home. Thank you to my sister, Margaret, and her husband, Wendell, for that first trip through Nine Mile Pond and for all the other adventures. And most important, I am deeply grateful to my husband, Gary, and sons, David and Jonathan. I could not have completed this project without your love and support.

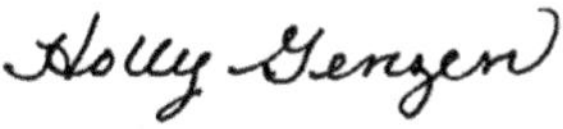

August 2011

I am grateful for the support of far and near friends, especially Karen, who has followed every paddling trip closely and aspires to paddling the Waterway herself someday.

Neighbors Mary and Jerry have watched the house during my paddling absences, calling sometimes while I was away just to check, "Are you OK?" And Norm, across the street, has helped with loading my 17.5-foot touring canoe on top of the car.

Most of all, I would like to thank my marine biologist mother, Dr. Anne McCrary, who taught me when I was very young how to manage a paddle and maneuver a small boat. Even more important, she taught me to love being out there.

And appreciation goes to my sons, Kenyata and Jolyon, who have learned to accept that there's just no telling what Mom is going to do next. I texted Jolyon from Sunday Bay one winter evening when Holly and I were stuck in mud and preparing to spend the night in the canoe; he texted back, "Mom, your life is 1 big adventure!" It is.

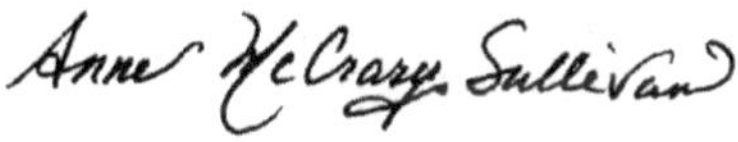

August 2011

Highland Beach Campsite

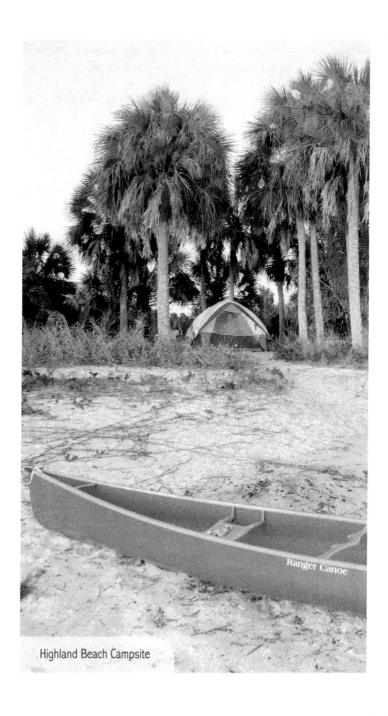

Preface

This guidebook is the one we wished we had on our first Waterway thru-paddle, when we carried copies of William G. Truesdell's *A Guide to the Wilderness Waterway of the Everglades National Park* (now out of print), along with selected pages from various guidebooks, pieced-together advice from park brochures and Internet resources, and a small library of books about the natural and social history of the Everglades. That was a fabulous trip, one that hooked us on the Waterway forever.

As we paddled, however, we grew in our belief that what was needed was a guidebook that offered comprehensive information about the practical aspects of paddling the Wilderness Waterway, one that also offered substantial but compact information about the natural and social history of the areas through which we traveled. We wanted a guidebook that included information about gear, safety, provisions, and planning; that provided ample maps with route descriptions; and that would still be good reading in the tent at night—so we wouldn't have to carry a library. We set out to write the book we wanted.

Marjory Stoneman Douglas began her 1947 classic, *The Everglades: River of Grass,* with the words, "There are no other Everglades in the world." We have found that canoeing and kayaking give you perspectives on Everglades National Park that you simply cannot get on land. Over time, as we have worked on this book, we have deepened our understanding of this magical place by undertaking repeated thru-paddles of the Everglades Wilderness Waterway, by exploring the 10,000 Islands and the Gulf of Mexico, by paddling canoe trails along old canals and airboat paths in the southern portion, and by dipping into the blue-green waters of Florida Bay. As Zora Neale Hurston writes in *Their Eyes Were Watching God,* "You got tuh *go* there tuh *know* there." Little by little, we have paddled our way to knowing there, but it's never enough; there's always more to know. We are always eager to get back out there.

We have experienced moments of unforgettable beauty: seeing the wash of stars spilling over the sky far from the city lights of Miami, gazing at flocks of ibis sweeping upriver at the end of the day to roost together in the mangroves, peering into pale-green beds of seagrass swaying beneath our boat and under the chickees in Florida Bay, watching stunning orange sunsets on the Gulf of Mexico, listening to barred owls calling throughout the night, observing the iridescent sheen of comb jellies in Alligator Creek, and glimpsing the pink of roseate spoonbills feeding in Garfield Bight.

We have been touched by remaining traces of human history: the writing on the cistern at Lopez River Campsite, the banana and avocado trees at Canepatch Campsite, the intricate shell mounds constructed by the early Native American Calusa people, the rusting farm equipment and the sugarcane kettle at The Watson Place, and what is now officially named Historic Smallwood Store.

Paddling, we have navigated high waves at the southeastern end of the Joe River, fought the incoming tide as we headed out to the Gulf of Mexico down Indian Key Pass, bumped into mangroves in the tight and twisting Noble Hammock Canoe Trail, and watched a pelican descend and *almost* land on our boat on the Broad River. At the end of the day, we have tied our canoe to mangroves and spent the night rocked to sleep by gentle waves.

The campsites brought their own memories: watching a habituated alligator watching *us* at Shark River Chickee, being visited by a manatee at Sweetwater Chickee, spotting the green flash at Highland Beach, slipping on marl at Alligator Creek Campsite, riding out a storm at Jewell Key, poking through tide-pools at Picnic Key, and lifting gear up onto the new tall chickees in Florida Bay.

You will form your own memories as you paddle through these waters. We hope that you enjoy these journeys as much as we have.

Happy paddling!

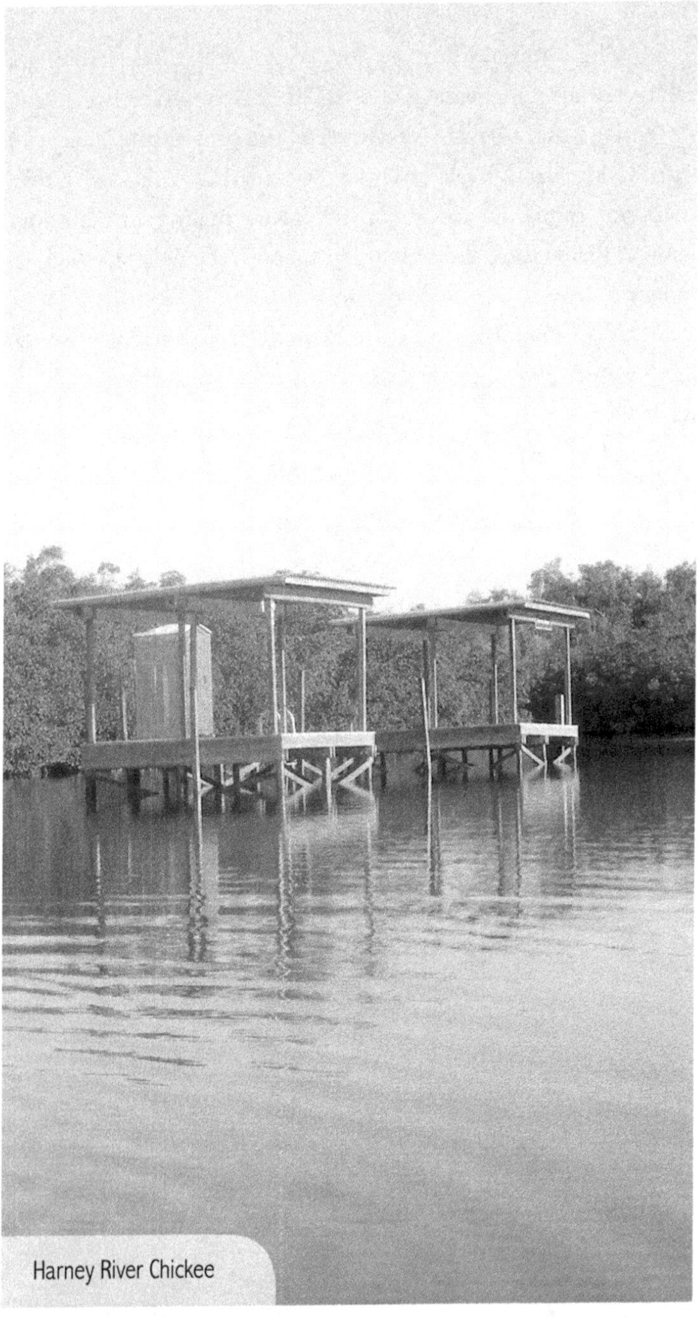

Harney River Chickee

Introduction

USING THIS GUIDE

Divided into six parts, this guidebook is designed for planning your Everglades trips and for use in conjunction with navigational charts while you are paddling.

Part One leads you on a thru-paddle of the Everglades Wilderness Waterway, with detailed information for trip preparation. The thru-paddle itinerary is presented in 21 sections of text, with 21 full-page maps juxtaposed for your convenience. The maps guide you both north to south and south to north between the put-in and takeout points in Everglades City and Flamingo. (Map 22, The Historical Route, presents the original, though not recommended, passage across Whitewater Bay.)

Part Two describes day and overnight paddles (with suggested campsites) in the north end of Everglades National Park. Each of those paddles launches from and returns to Everglades City. No shuttles are required.

Part Three guides you on day and overnight paddles (and suggested campsites) in the south end of the park, launching from either the park road west of Homestead or from Flamingo. As with the trips from Everglades City, no shuttles are required.

In both Parts Two and Three, we open each day trip or overnight excursion with an overview of six key items:

- the waterway or destination name
- distance in miles

- estimated paddle time in hours
- potential hazards
- GPS coordinates for significant points on that route
- navigational references

Then we provide a brief description of each route and a run profile with commentary on the human history and flora and fauna of the area. Regarding the paddling duration given for these day and overnight trips, all times are approximate, depending on several factors: your paddling speed, whether you are moving with or against the tides, and, not to be overlooked, the number and length of breaks and photo stops along the way.

The potential hazards we cite in the overviews in Parts Two and Three include oyster beds, mudflats, strong currents, and other tide-related occurrences; wind and waves in open water; heavy boat traffic; wet and dry cycles; and hurricane season. (But we will remind you here and elsewhere to always check with the visitor centers for current conditions on your chosen routes.)

Part Four describes the particular challenges of summertime paddling in the Everglades.

Part Five describes the campsites that are cross-referenced in the Wilderness Waterway section (Part One) and in the overnight descriptions (Parts Two and Three).

Part Six provides interesting information about the natural and social history that will become part of your Everglades experience.

THE MAPS

The maps in this guidebook show put-in and takeout points; campsite locations; navigational markers; historical sites; and significant islands, bays, and streams. While these maps are exceedingly helpful to you as you plan and paddle the routes, do not rely solely on them for navigation. You will be traveling through intricate interlacings of mangrove islands and waterways. *For safety's sake, you must carry navigational charts if you undertake the full Everglades Wilderness Waterway.* Charts are not as necessary for day trips, although they are always helpful as an extra precaution.

ROUTE DESCRIPTIONS

For the grand, 99-mile journey along the full length of the Everglades Wilderness Waterway, or even for a significant portion of it, the location of campsites and route paddling conditions described in this guide will help you determine an appropriate itinerary. Run profiles for short paddles from Everglades City or Flamingo offer choices; some lead you into the wilderness, and some keep you closer to civilization. Either way, you'll find paddles for varying skill levels and interests.

GPS COORDINATES

We used a Global Positioning System (GPS) receiver to pinpoint the coordinates, or intersection of latitude and longitude lines, along each route or at each destination referenced throughout this book. For example, the box on the next page depicts the location of the beginning and end of the single Wilderness Waterway section we have labeled 1/U. (Sections in this guidebook are numbered 1–21 for the north-to-south route and lettered A–U for the south-to-north route, and all GPS coordinates are presented in the degree–decimal minute format.)

For a complete list of the GPS waypoints for the Wilderness Waterway, see Appendix 7, Everglades Wilderness Waterway GPS Coordinates, on page 288.

The latitude and longitude grid system is likely quite familiar to you, but here is a refresher, pertinent to visualizing the GPS coordinates.

Imaginary lines of latitude—called parallels and approximately 69 miles apart from each other—run horizontally around the globe. Each parallel is indicated by degrees from the equator (established to be 0°): up to 90°N at the North Pole, and down to 90°S at the South Pole.

Imaginary lines of longitude—called meridians—run perpendicular to latitude lines. Longitude lines are likewise indicated by degrees: starting from 0° at the Prime Meridian in Greenwich, England, they continue to the east and west until they meet 180° later at the International Date Line in the Pacific Ocean. At the equator, longitude lines also are approximately 69 miles apart, but that distance narrows as the meridians converge toward the North and South poles.

To convert GPS coordinates given in degrees, minutes, and seconds to the format shown in the box below—degrees–decimal minutes, simply divide the seconds by 60.

For more on GPS technology, visit **usgs.gov.**

GPS Coordinates

SECTION 1/U: EVERGLADES CITY (GULF COAST VISITOR CENTER)/ CHOKOLOSKEE ISLAND (SOUTH END)

Gulf Coast Visitor Center: N25° 50.730′ W81° 23.234′
Chokoloskee Island: N25° 48.537′ W81° 21.442′

CHARTS & USGS QUADRANGLES

At Everglades visitor centers, you can get maps for a few of the popular routes, such as Sandfly Island in the north and Nine Mile Pond and Hells Bay Canoe Trail in the south. Otherwise, for most of the paddles described in this book, navigational charts are essential. (See "Navigation" on page 36, and resources for buying the charts in Appendix 2, Launch Sites, page 269, and Appendix 5, Internet Sources, page 281.)

When you paddle interior routes not covered by nautical charts, the U.S. Geological Survey (USGS) 7.5-minute quadrangles (**usgs.gov/pub**) are useful (see page 283). We list the quads in the overview information for each of those routes.

SHUTTLE DIRECTIONS

The Wilderness Waterway thru-paddle section of this guidebook includes shuttle information. Outfitters offering shuttle service are listed in Appendix 4, Resource Overview, on page 278. All other paddles described in this guidebook start and end at the same location, so shuttles are not necessary.

PARKING & SECURING YOUR VEHICLE

When launching from Gulf Coast Visitor Center in the north or from Flamingo Visitor Center in the south, you may leave your car in the parking areas by the launch site. If you plan to paddle one of the canoe trails off the main park road in the southern section of the park, you will find a small parking area near your put-in. Either way, secure your valuables and lock your car.

When you make backcountry campsite reservations, you will need to provide your vehicle license plate number, but there is no charge for use of the National Park Service (NPS) parking areas. (*Note:* It is understood that your car may be parked for more than a week if you paddle the entire Wilderness Waterway.)

PADDLING CONDITIONS

This section provides an overview of what to expect and plan for when you undertake your Everglades adventure.

MEAN WATER TEMPERATURES BY MONTH

Typically, water temperature is not a big issue for Everglades paddlers (though it is for fishermen). However, it is good to know that the National Oceanic and Atmospheric Administration (NOAA) site **nodc.noaa.gov/dsdt** shows water-temperature fluctuations for the region throughout the seasons. In July and August, the water temperature can reach into the high 80s; when a cold front comes through in the winter, the temperature can drop to the low 60s. To find current water-temperature data, you can access **wunderground.com/MAR/GM/676** or **marine.rutgers.edu/cool/sat_data.**

GAUGING WATER LEVELS

The water-monitoring stations that you pass as you paddle in the Everglades measure water conditions such as temperature, flow, salinity, and water quality. This information is sent via satellite to the USGS. Its website **waterdata.usgs.gov/nwis/rt** traces the twice-daily rise and fall of water level and salinity, clearly showing how waterways in the Everglades are influenced by tides.

In addition to the daily tidal changes in water level, the yearly cycles of the rainy season (April–October) and dry season (November–March) affect many of your trips through the Everglades. In the dry season, there is a foot less water in the entire system than in the rainy season. A dry-season low tide may cause some routes to be impassable and make some chickees (sleeping platforms) inaccessible. Still, many of the routes in this guidebook are navigable in both wet and dry seasons. If a route or campsite might be difficult or impossible to access in dry conditions, we make note of this. But we suggest that you always inquire about current conditions at the visitor center.

The National Park Service (NPS) is the best source for current information about water levels on particular routes or campsites. For conditions at the north end of the park, call the Gulf Coast Visitor Center at (239) 695-3311; for the south end of the park, call the Flamingo Visitor Center at (239) 695-2945.

MIND THE TIDES

Keep in mind that one moderate low tide is generally followed by a high tide and then a more extensive low tide. But your awareness of the tides is more important in some areas than others. (See "Navigation" on page 36.) When paddling routes closely connected to the Gulf of Mexico, tide information is essential. Before leaving home, always download a tide chart (see **saltwatertides.com**), or ask for a tide chart at the visitor center. Paddling against the tide can double the time and effort required for some trips, so in the overview information that introduces each paddle in this book, we indicate the routes where it is particularly important to check tide tables.

A WORD ABOUT BOATING SKILLS

For safety's sake, know your abilities on the water. If you are a beginner, choose day trips from the park's north (see page 118) or south (see page 154) routes, or one-nighters on the Wilderness Waterway, before attempting to paddle longer segments of the Waterway. Trails such as Nine Mile Pond or the Buttonwood Canal minimize the dangers of wind and waves, while at the same time exposing you to the richness of Everglades bird life and vegetation. Kayakers and canoeists with more experience in paddling and navigation might choose longer trips through the rivers and bays in the Glades. Veteran paddlers can tackle the full Wilderness Waterway experience.

WATERWAY HAZARDS & SAFETY

While the Everglades may seem forbidding to absolute beginners, novices can enjoy some of the routes described in this guidebook. For all the pleasures, there are risks to consider when you head out onto any body of water, and paddling the Everglades is no exception. You may encounter waves caused by windy conditions in the bays and the Gulf of Mexico; strong tidal flow in rivers close to the Gulf; shallow water with exposed oyster beds, seagrass meadows, and mudflats; and mangrove tangles in narrow passages.

Paddlers may face heavy powerboat traffic on some routes, especially in high season. In every season in this part of the country, there is the risk of sunburn and heatstroke. Summer brings volatile thunderstorms, and winter introduces the chance of hypothermia. We highlight particular hazards of the routes in the introductory material for each route and give more detailed safety information in Parts One and Four, pages 26 and 201, respectively.

EMERGENCY RESCUE

Everglades paddlers often travel in remote areas, especially if you follow the entire Wilderness Waterway. While isolation adds to the beauty and appeal of the Everglades, there are no roadways where you will be paddling. Thus, any rescue along the routes covered in this guidebook will be by boat or helicopter.

If you find yourself in an emergency situation, stay with your boat and, if possible, remain near a marker or a campsite. Most of the Everglades National Park paddling area does not have cell phone coverage. For the full Waterway trip, we recommend carrying a marine radio, both for weather reports and to call for help in emergencies. The U.S. Coast Guard monitors channel 16, and powerboaters are required to keep their radios on and tuned to channel 16 to report emergency calls coming over the radio. Some paddlers may want to invest in or rent a satellite phone or a personal locator beacon, known as a PLB.

Still, never depend on electronic equipment alone. Trip planning and preparation, maps, a compass, and navigation skills should always be a part of paddling in this water world. Be sure to monitor weather reports in advance and check at the visitor center for seasonal conditions. Always carry more water than you think you will need, as well as extra food, emergency supplies, and first-aid equipment.

When paddling the Waterway or any of the overnight routes in this guidebook, you must make campsite reservations in person at one of the visitor centers within 24 hours before your launch, but you will not be required to check out when you complete the trip. Thus, prior to launching, be sure to let someone know your itinerary and give that person the park's emergency number: (305) 242-7740.

For more information on safety, see page 38, and for more on equipment, see pages 42 and 44. Also see Appendix 1, Checklist, on page 266.

WEATHER BY SEASON

Generally, Florida's sunshine and warm temperatures make it an ideal destination for year-round paddling, as long as seasonal conditions are taken into account. Save the full Wilderness Waterway trip for fall, winter, or spring to avoid thunderstorms, extreme heat, and myriad insects. In the summertime, explore breezy, beautiful Chokoloskee Bay, do the serene Hurddles Creek Loop, or head out toward the Gulf of Mexico or Florida Bay, where the wind can blow the bugs away. Regardless of season, take along plenty of sunscreen, insect repellent, and water.

Winter

The region's dry winter season—with clear skies, lower temperatures, and fewer mosquitoes and biting flies—is the most popular time for paddling. Temperatures average a daily high in the upper 70s and lows in the upper 50s. Monthly precipitation averages below 2 inches. But be aware that cold fronts may come through, dropping temperatures into the 30s and 40s. Cold fronts also can bring north winds that sweep water out of small bays, making some routes and campsites difficult to access. Be sure to check at the visitor centers for up-to-the-minute weather conditions.

Spring

The moderate temperatures and low rainfall of an Everglades spring begin in February and run into May. Spring highs average in the 80s in the daytime, 60s at night. Rainfall averages around 2 inches, increasing to 5 inches as the rainy season begins. A disadvantage of springtime paddling is that it comes at the end of the dry season. Water levels may still be low, creating more extensive mudflats and exposed oyster beds in tidal areas and making some interior routes too shallow to paddle.

Summer

This is the rainy season, with higher water levels caused by daily afternoon thunderstorms and the occasional tropical storm or hurricane. Rainfall averages for the summer range from just below 5 inches in July to more than 7.5 inches in August. Average temperatures run from the high 80s and low 90s in the daytime to the mid-70s at night. Mosquitoes and biting flies are much more of a nuisance this time of year, so be sure to protect yourself with insect repellent and/or bug suits. On the positive side, summertime paddling on short routes brings great opportunities for wildlife viewing and for a quiet, uncrowded experience. (See Part Four, Summer Paddling, on page 201.)

Fall

In October and November, the extreme heat of summer is over, and the threat of afternoon thunderstorms has receded. Fall temperatures may hit the 80s in the daytime but drop to the 60s and 70s at night. Fall rainfall averages 4.25 inches in October, decreasing to 2.5 inches in November as you move into the dry season. And because rains have been falling for several months, there's more water in the system. Paddling is lovely. But watch weather reports for afternoon thunderstorms or approaching tropical storms.

WILDLIFE

Birds

We present the topic of Everglades birds within the broader context of the Everglades ecology and environment (see page 18).

Insects

These invertebrates are the smallest and least appreciated of the wildlife you will encounter in the Everglades. The most bothersome are mosquitoes, known as "swamp angels"; no-see-ums, also called sand flies; and yellow flies, often referred to as deer flies. At certain times of the year and in some locations, biting insects can be fierce, so bring plenty of insect repellent and be sure to have a tent with fine-mesh netting. Carry some topical Benadryl or other remedy to soothe your itches after the inevitable bites. (For additional tips on dealing with nuisance insects, see "Insects" on page 204.)

You also may hear the buzz of black-and-yellow mud daubers, which are nonaggressive wasps that build tubular mud nests under chickee roofs. Less frequently encountered are paper wasps, whose nests may be found hanging from branches over narrow passages. Although these wasps are not aggressive either, take care not to knock the nest with your kayak paddle. They *will* defend their nest from attack.

But don't forget to notice the charms of smaller wildlife. You may feel more welcoming toward other insects—especially the beautiful ones without stingers. We marvel at the butterflies that flutter around our boat far out on open water; at the large, patterned moths at the chickees; and at the dragonflies in the mangroves when we tie up for lunch or wait out a storm.

Mammals

There is little chance of seeing a bear or Florida panther in the Everglades any longer, although you may spot a bobcat. We have seen bats at several campsites and know there are opossums in the Everglades because Darwin's Place is on Opossum Key. But we have never seen opossums, bears, or panthers.

Raccoons, however, are a different story. As smart and aggressive in the Everglades as they are elsewhere, raccoons will try to steal your food at ground sites, so be sure to secure your food supply with bungee cords. And because freshwater is scarce in the Glades, they may also try to chew their way into your water containers. Although we have never had problems with rats, the park rangers have related stories of these critters being pesky at campsites too. As long as you protect your supplies, however, seeing raccoons and rats can be part of the adventure.

You might catch a glimpse of deer, particularly if you stay at Highland Beach. Although deer are generally upland creatures, even antlered deer can penetrate the thick tangle of mangrove forests.

But the most frequent mammals you will encounter on your paddles are Atlantic bottlenose dolphins. Although they are saltwater mammals, dolphins travel upriver in search of prey and can be observed splashing in bays or herding fish onto riverbanks. They are curious and sometimes tilt their bodies to watch you with an inquisitive eye.

Consider yourself fortunate if you encounter another marine mammal, the manatee. Not carnivorous like dolphins, manatees feed on seagrass and can be spotted at the mouths of Everglades rivers or in the Flamingo marina. Look for manatee

Dolphin splash

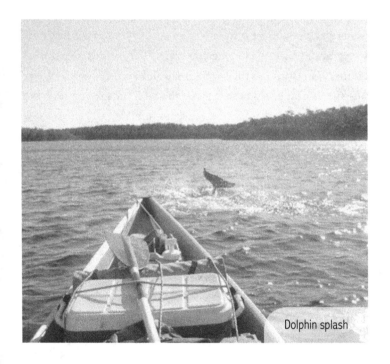

"footprints," the flat circles on the surface of the water that indicate a manatee may be paddling by.

Oysters

This may surprise you, but one animal of the Everglades that has the potential to cause harm is the oyster. This marine invertebrate starts its life in larval form floating around in salt water until it anchors itself with many other oyster larvae on a shallow spit of land. There it makes its living filtering food from the incoming tide. The danger lies in the fact that oyster shells are razor-sharp and some oysters carry disease—*Vibrio vulnificus* or *Vibrio parahaemolyticus*. To avoid cuts, we advise you to always wear water shoes while paddling—and do not step out of your boat without those shoes securely on your feet.

Reptiles

Many people who venture into the Everglades for the first time worry about snakes and alligators. We've seen only two snakes on the Waterway and they were small and nonvenomous. We're sure there must be some snakes out there on the ground sites, but snakes tend to want to keep away from humans.

Widespread press coverage of nonnative pythons, introduced into the park by pet-owner release, may raise questions for some. These pythons are reproducing, and the population of small mammals, a food source, seems to be diminishing. Park biologists are studying these reptiles, and they ask that anyone who sees a python notify them of the location.

As you paddle, you may see alligators on the banks along the routes, but these animals are shy and will slide into the water as you pass. The only cases where we have observed this not to be the case is when an alligator hangs around a campsite because it has become habituated to getting scraps from campers and

Alligator on the Broad River

fishermen. When fed by humans, alligators can become dangerous. So do not dump food scraps, even small ones, into the water.

American crocodiles also have a presence in the Glades. They are an endangered species, and you will be fortunate if you see one, with its pointed snout and toothy grin. Whereas alligators prefer fresh or brackish water, American crocodiles require salt or brackish water. Like the alligator, the American crocodile is a nonthreatening presence in its natural habitat. Enjoy these creatures respectfully.

For more on individual members of the animal kingdom, see Part Six, Everglades Flora, Fauna, People, & Places, on page 243.

CAMPING

Two front-country, drive-in campgrounds sit at the southeastern entrance to the park near Homestead. Long Pine Key

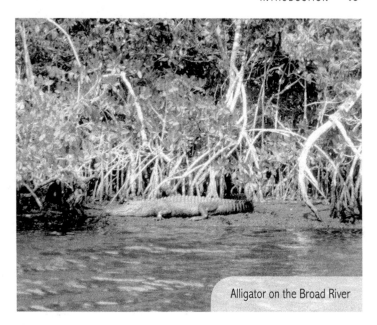

Campground, which *does not* accept reservations, is 6 miles southwest of the Ernest F. Coe Visitor Center. Flamingo Campground, which *does* take reservations, is on Florida Bay, near the Flamingo Visitor Center at the end of the 38-mile park road. (Additional lodging and campgrounds are available near the northern and southern ends of Everglades National Park and are listed in Appendix 4, Resource Overview, on page 278.)

You must make reservations with the NPS to camp at any of the three types of backcountry sites available within the park and briefly described here. For detailed information about each overnight locale referenced in this book, please see Part Five, The Campsites, on page 213. Also visit **nps.gov/ever**.

Chickees

Constructed on pilings over water, chickees are open-sided, wooden platforms with a roof. See more about chickees on page 32, in "Camping on Water, Land, & Shore."

Ground Sites

Ground sites consist of small, cleared areas primarily on old Calusa shell mounds. Most ground sites have picnic tables and portable toilets, and some have docks.

Beach Sites

Beach sites are just what their name suggests—campsites directly on the sandy shores of the Gulf of Mexico or on keys in Florida Bay.

YOUR RIGHTS & RESPONSIBILITIES

The paddles described in this book are all within Everglades National Park, whose waters have been preserved from development and commercial use by the NPS. As members of the public, we are invited to enter the Glades thoughtfully and responsibly. An entrance fee is required for access at the south end (Homestead) and, except in the summertime, you must also pay a small fee for a permit if you intend to camp.

Rules and regulations are printed on Everglades camping permits and in the Wilderness Trip Planner brochure available at the visitor centers or online at **nps.gov/ever.** When you purchase permits, a ranger will go over the requirements. Examples of regulations include:

- Florida Bay keys are closed for boat landings (except for Bradley Key and the keys designated as campsites).
- Access to some islands and bays is limited because of protected bird rookeries.
- Fires are *not* permitted except on beach sites.
- No ash-producing fuel, such as charcoal or wood, may be used on chickees or ground sites.
- Leave no trace. Whatever you take with you, you must pack out.
- Urinate directly into the water; for human waste, if there is no privy, bury the matter 6 inches deep in the ground.

The areas immediately around Everglades City and Chokoloskee Island are not themselves part of Everglades National Park. When visiting or launching from these sites, please respect landowners' rights. Be aware, as well, that many of the outfitters and marina operators in this area are descendants of original pioneer families. They are knowledgeable and proud of where they live, and they will be helpful to and appreciative of those who respect the history and the ecological integrity of their home. Many of the residents are committed to offering ecotourism opportunities. We encourage you to get to know them if you have questions or need guides.

WATERWAY ETIQUETTE

Here are a few reminders to enhance everyone's pleasure:

- Stay to the side of channels and, if motorboaters slow to idle speed, stop paddling until they pass. To avoid being swamped when powerboats pass without slowing, turn your bow into the wake.
- For group paddles, plan your choice of campsites carefully. Only one tent will fit on a single chickee platform (double chickees accommodate two), and ground sites as well as some beach sites are small. For the maximum number of people and parties allowed at each location, see Part Five, The Campsites, on page 213. And remember, unless you encounter dangerous conditions or emergency situations, do not stay at sites you have not reserved.
- When camping in proximity to others, be respectful of their needs for a quiet and peaceful wilderness experience.

ECOLOGY & ENVIRONMENT

Diverse waters mingle in the Everglades. The Wilderness Waterway and the paddling areas to the north and south of it are fed by three different watersheds, each of which is called a slough (pronounced "slew"). Here is a brief orientation:

When you are deep in wilderness in the central areas of the Waterway, you will be paddling in waters from the Shark River Slough as it travels to the Gulf of Mexico.

When you travel routes in the Chokoloskee Bay area, you are paddling in water of the Fakahatchee Slough, which has passed through Big Cypress Swamp.

If you paddle one of the canoe trails off the park road at the south end of Everglades National Park, you will be traveling on water from Taylor Slough.

And if you venture out into Florida Bay, you leave the freshwater flow of the sloughs behind and enter an open marine environment spreading from the tip of peninsular Florida to the Florida Keys.

THIS "RIVER OF GRASS"

The definition of the word Everglades is unknown, although the term may have its roots in the Middle English word *glad,* meaning "bright, shining." The venerable author, environmentalist, and Everglades champion Marjorie Stoneman Douglas (1890–1998) aptly called her beloved wetlands and her 1947 classic work, *The Everglades: River of Grass.* In that book (a 60th-anniversary edition was published in 2007), she noted that the term Everglades first appeared on an 1823 map.

Seminoles called it *Pa-hay-okee,* meaning "grassy water." In his account of his 1896–97 trip, *Across the Everglades*, Hugh Willoughby described it as "a sea of apparently pathless grass." Naturalist author Ted Levin titled his Everglades book *Liquid Land.*

Regardless of the word's source, these "glad" Glades, this bright, shining place, consists of 1,508,571 acres that stretch diagonally from the southern Gulf Coast of Florida into Florida Bay. The region's aesthetic and ecological value has earned it three of our planet's most prominent designations: International Biosphere Reserve, a World Heritage Site, and a Wetland of International Significance.

All appellations aside, the place is surprising. Visitors often expect to see swamps and cypress trees and are awed by the sawgrass prairies extending across a flat landscape to the horizon. In fact, the Everglades harbors five distinct ecosystems:

- sawgrass prairie
- hardwood hammock
- mangrove forest
- rock pineland
- dwarf cypress forest

While most of the paddling areas are in the mangroves, if you enter the park on the Homestead side and drive the 38 miles of the main park road to Flamingo, you will pass through all five ecosystems. In that short distance, you will travel from freshwater sawgrass through brackish habitats to saline estuaries characterized by mangroves.

With its mosaic of habitats, a unique combination of geography, water flow, and weather, the Everglades presents an ideal environment for a rich diversity of both plants and animals. Poised at both the southern limit of the temperate zone and the northern limit for many tropical species, temperate and tropical species blend here in ways that are rare in the world. It is this richness of biological diversity that earned the Everglades its status as a national park. This was the first park to be preserved not for its gigantic or geological wonders but for its biological uniqueness and the subtleties of its cycles.

WADING BIRDS

Because these flying creatures are such an encompassing part of Everglades environment and history, as well as an indicator for its future, we include them in this discussion rather than in the previous "Wildlife" section.

In the wondrous diversity of the Everglades, wading birds are among the features people most admire and enjoy. Wood storks, white ibis, glossy ibis, and roseate spoonbills soar over the park's wetlands. Herons and egrets of all sorts—great blue, little blue, green, reddish, and tricolored herons and great and snowy egrets—wade and wait along narrow streams, in shallow seagrass meadows, and on low-tide mudflats. But there are not as many as there once were.

Nothing was more striking at one time than the vast numbers of wading birds that fed and multiplied in the Everglades. Audubon wardens in the 1930s estimated a population of 250,000 wading birds, primarily white ibis, along with roseate spoonbills, egrets, herons, and wood storks. But that population was small compared to the sightings of earlier naturalists. They wrote of flocks that blackened the sky. For decades, dating back into the early 1800s, the beauty of these birds' nuptial plumage charmed not only potential mates and Florida naturalists but also the eye of big-city fashion designers who sought to adorn ladies' hats with feathers. There was money to be made as a plumer, with the price of feathers rising to $32 an ounce (which would equal almost $800 an ounce today).

As the feather trend raged, the population of wading birds was being decimated, with hunters often shooting up an entire rookery, killing hundreds or even thousands of adult birds on the nest, leaving eggs and chicks abandoned. Finally, in 1901 the state of Florida passed Chapter 4357, a bird protection act that opened the way for game wardens to patrol the rookeries in the Everglades. Contracted by the American Ornithologists' Union (which later became the Audubon Society), Guy Bradley was the first of these wardens. He was killed in 1905 when he went after suspected plume hunters in the Oyster Keys of Florida Bay. Bradley was the first of several wardens who would lose their lives in the line of duty. (For more on Guy Bradley, see the Johnson Key overnight paddle description, on page 183.)

Ultimately, it was fashionable women themselves who came to the rescue of the birds. For a while they had believed what they were told, that the birds shed their feathers naturally. When the truth came to light, small groups of women banded together to boycott and to urge others to boycott hats that were adorned with feathers. As fashion changed and demand dropped, so did the price paid to plumers for feathers, and the trade ceased to be profitable.

Since then, bird populations have recovered somewhat, but issues related to water quality, quantity, and timing have interfered with a fuller recovery. For decades, discussions of how to preserve what remains of the Glades, its birds, and other biological wonders have circled, repeated, and droned on, as funds for restoration have been allocated and then never delivered and as life-giving water dynamics have deteriorated.

Sometimes, for example, large quantities of water have been unnaturally released into the park from dikes built to protect agricultural lands and developments. Such a release of water, at a time when water levels in the park would normally be low, can have devastating effects on wildlife, including the endangered wood stork, the only true stork native to North America. These birds are touch feeders: they locate their prey by moving their curved beaks in shallow water until the beak bumps into something, at which point it opens and snaps up whatever fish or crustacean it has bumped. During the nesting season, a wood stork needs to have several hundred pounds of nourishment, an ounce or two at a time, bump into its beak in order to have sufficient food for itself and its young. Shallow water, where creatures are concentrated, is essential. If water comes roaring in from the north during the wood stork's nesting time, artificially raising water levels and dispersing aquatic animals, the stork cannot feed its young, and a whole nesting season, for a bird already endangered, can be lost. Water timing is essential. The dry season is as life-supporting as the wet season.

For more on the prevalent bird species you are apt to observe here, see Part Six, Everglades Flora, Fauna, People, & Places, on page 243.

EVERGLADES UNDER THREAT

We will never see what the original vast expanse of sawgrass must have been like. Agriculture, urban expansion, and dredging have forever altered natural Florida. The full Everglades system, stretching from just south of Orlando to Florida Bay, is now beyond the possibility of restoration. Everglades National Park protects only about one-fifth of the original Everglades, and even this fraction is endangered.

The Everglades formed approximately 5,000 years ago when rain and rising sea levels flooded South Florida. Natural barriers formed by the Atlantic Coastal Ridge on the east and, to a lesser extent, Big Cypress Swamp on the west held these waters in a shallow trough, forcing them to make a journey south from Lake Okeechobee to the tip of the Florida peninsula. In this flow, upland plant species died, and marsh plants such as Jamaica swamp sawgrass *(Cladium jamaicense)* thrived, becoming the primary vegetation of the "River of Grass."

Waters of these historical Everglades originated in central Florida in the Kissimmee River. Fed by drenching summer rains, river waters flowed slowly southward toward the shallow, southward-tilting bowl of Lake Okeechobee. Spilling over the edges of Okeechobee, the wide, shallow flow continued ("an excruciatingly slow descent," according to author Archie Carr) in two directions—southwest to the Gulf of Mexico and south into Florida Bay.

But in 1904, a time when most of South Florida was viewed as useless swampland, Governor Napoleon Bonaparte Broward campaigned under the slogan "Drain the Everglades," and the land boom began. The areas south of Lake Okeechobee buzzed and clattered with activity—dredging canals to drain the land and irrigate fields for sugarcane, vegetable farming, and ranching industries; building roads; and constructing housing developments. The Everglades, whose area once totaled 6,000 square miles, began to dry up. Canals and construction interrupted the flow and threatened ecosystems that would become increasingly dependent upon rainfall as a source of water.

Wood stork

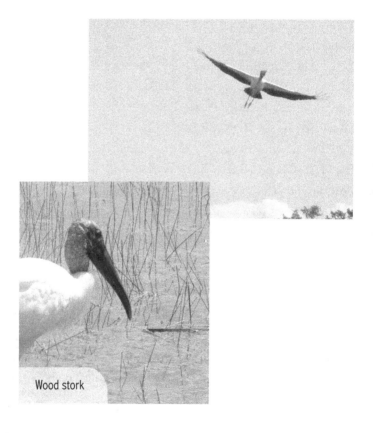

Although the dominant cultural idea of the time was to drain and develop, some people recognized that a rich resource was being lost. In 1916 the Florida Federation of Women's Clubs lobbied to preserve a small portion of land in the Glades, a hammock called Royal Palm. Then, along with similar groups and noteworthy individuals such as Ernest F. Coe and Marjory Stoneman Douglas, they labored over the next 30 years promoting the creation of a national park. In 1947, with neither spectacular mountain scenery nor dramatic waterfalls and canyons, Everglades National Park became the first national park established to protect plants and animals and their unique habitat. But protection hasn't been easy because the park is affected by what happens outside its boundaries. Water that does get through to the Glades from the north, either naturally or by human decision, is often polluted by runoff.

But all of the news is not bad. One major, long-awaited project has broken ground—a stretch of bridge to replace a section of the Tamiami Trail (FL 41), a road that has, in effect, been damming the flow of water into the Everglades. This bridge is hailed as an essential element in assuring that the ecosystems of the park can survive.

Further Information

*For information and updates on threats to the Everglades and current preservation and restoration efforts, including how you can help, consult the websites of Friends of the Everglades (***everglades.org***), an organization founded in 1969 by Marjory Stoneman Douglas, and Audubon of Florida (***fl.audubon.org***).*

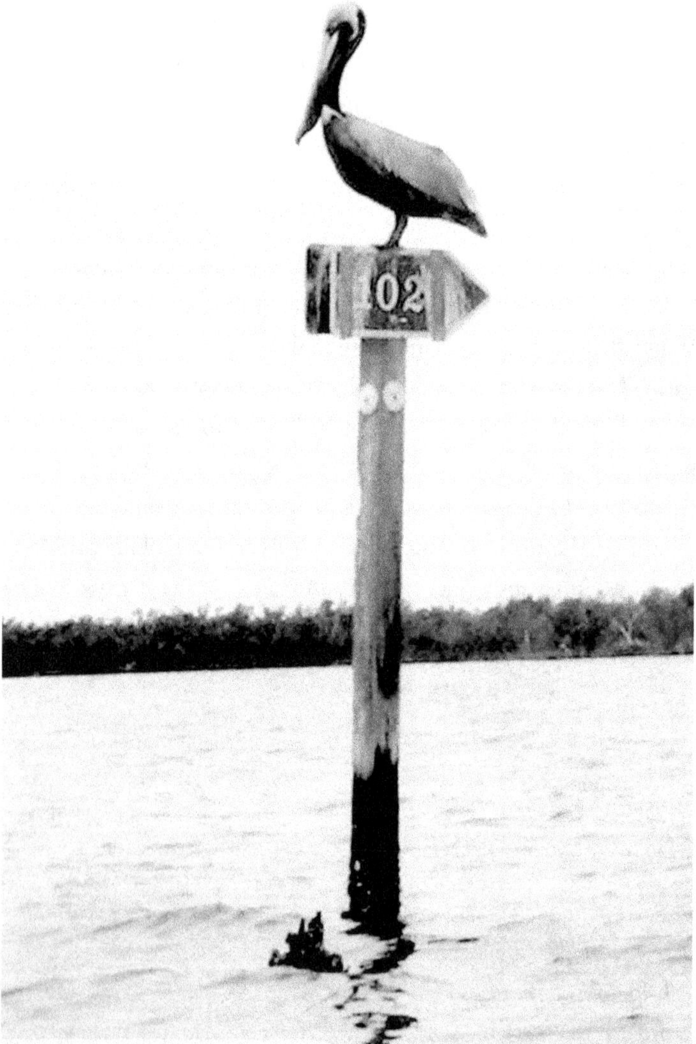

Brown pelican on marker 102

Part One:

On the Everglades Wilderness Waterway

MEET THE WATERWAY

Mapped in the mid-1960s, the Everglades Wilderness Waterway is a 99-mile-long trail of bays, channels, and rivers that makes it possible to travel inland by water from Everglades City, at the northwestern edge of the park, southeast to Flamingo on Florida Bay. Paddling this route delivers you back into the world of the people living in the Glades before the park was created in 1947. You will have a sense of what it was like for early Native Americans, the Calusa, who passed among shell mounds and middens, sustaining themselves with the bounty of the sea, and later, the Seminoles, who traveled to hide in the backcountry during the Seminole Wars. Paddling this inland route will also give you a feel for the lives of early pioneers who chose to avoid the open water of the Gulf during rough weather. More important, the interior offered them a place to hunt alligators for their hides, shoot birds for their plumes, and escape from the authorities as they made their living during hard times "moonshining" and carrying out other activities that were a shade below the law.

Think, for a moment, how it must have been for these Native Americans and early pioneers who could find the places you will learn of in this book without depending on charts or modern GPS. They could go to Sweetwater for freshwater, or to Smallwood's store to trade; to Watson's place to purchase corn syrup from the dreaded Mr. Watson (if they dared; see page 239); to Shark River to work in the tanning trade; or to the cistern at Lopez's or Darwin's if their own water was salted by storm tides. The Waterway was an early "highway" through the Glades. Those who traveled it knew the bays and creeks as well as you know the roads close to your own home. Taking this 99-mile trip will give you a feeling of being in their neighborhood, of reliving a part of history.

Expecting to navigate channels through sawgrass or passages in a cypress swamp, some may be surprised when heading out on the Waterway for the first time. The route winds through waters lined with mangroves—in wide or small bays, broad rivers, or narrow twisting channels—the red (*Rizophora mangle*), with their arching prop roots; the black (*Avicennia germinans*), with their pneumatophores; and the tall white (*Laguncularia racemosa*), rising above the canopy.

In the water or along the shore, posts with brown arrows and white numbers mark the Waterway. Whether you launch from Flamingo and count the letters up, or launch from Everglades City and count the numbers up, you are in for a fine adventure through wilderness and history.

HOW IT CAME TO BE

The idea of a marked waterway permitting small boats to make an inland passage from Everglades City to Flamingo was born in the 1950s. Daniel Beard, the first superintendent of Everglades National Park, included such a passage in his planning, but there was no known natural connector between the Broad River and the Shark River, and dredging would have damaged the ecosystem.

The idea lay dormant until the 1960s, when ranger Richard "Dick" Stokes began searching the charts for indications of a possible passage. In a December 12, 1996, open letter, he writes of his experiences laying out the route for the Waterway: "The first charts of this area were called T-Charts. They were in black and white with no depths on them. In studying these charts I found that there was a creek from Broad River into Broad Creek which went into the Harney River and thence to the Shark. . . . " These charts "showed three small creeks off the main creek which would make the connection."

Stokes began to plan for an attempt to locate these creeks, starting in August of 1966. Ranger Stokes, park superintendent Roger Allin, and chief ranger Bob Kerr searched for but failed to find a connecting channel. (For the story, see "The Nightmare," on page 256.) Soon after, Stokes returned with a small party to try again. His letter continues, "[W]e took the same route through the main creek, but this time we took the fourth creek instead of the third. With a little effort we made it through to Broad Creek. This was the first trip through the waterway."

"A little effort" is an understatement. The process of clearing this narrow, twisting channel that had filled up with storm debris would take months. Park archives indicate that in December 1967, five men spent four days cutting out Wood River Creek "with not much visible progress." In April of the following year, rangers were still making trips to assess how much more clearing needed to be done, but by May 1968, the route was described in administrative reports as "newly-cleared," although still with "submerged snags."

With this critical connecting piece somewhat in place, the process of formally laying out the route from Everglades City to Flamingo was possible, and then in midsummer heat, the actual installation of the markers began.

THE FIRST WATERWAY GUIDEBOOK

On January 15, 1967, transferring from Shenandoah National Park, in Virginia, ranger William G. Truesdell reported for duty in the Everglades and soon participated in officially marking the Wilderness Waterway. In a March 15, 2010, e-mail to the authors, he wrote, "Art Johnson, district ranger at Everglades City; Larry Dale, park ranger at Everglades City; Johnny Galvin, maintenance employee; and I put in the posts . . . in the middle of summer." He called up "memories of the flat barge loaded with 6-inch-by-6-inch-by-16-foot-long posts, using a water pressure pump to dig the posts in, and hot, humid days with lots of mosquitoes."

The placing of posts, he explains, was "determined primarily by the need to have a marker close enough to the previous one so that the boater didn't turn before the required turn. Not necessarily line-of-sight, but if two alternative routes came together at one point, a marker had to be placed on that point." They would place the post "just around the edge of the turn, as opposed to right on the corner" and "just far enough out in the channel to be visible." The positioning of the markers was completed by the middle of August 1968, when ranger Stokes and park superintendent Allin, who had made the first attempt to find a passage, completed a triumphant inspection run of the trail.

Meanwhile, Truesdell had begun drawing strip maps of the entire waterway, section by section, and writing text to accompany the maps in what he initially called a "handbook on the Mangrove Wilderness." In the text, he described critical places in the route and sketched notes on natural and social history. The project occupied him for another full year, as he carried out his other duties. At the same time he worked on numbering the markers that had already been placed along the trail.

In spring 1969, Truesdell reported that the *Guide to the Wilderness Waterway* had been "rewritten for the 'umpteenth' time and submitted to Miami Press" and that "every marker on the route has now been numbered." In September, that first guidebook, spiral-bound, with a green-tinted cover, was done. Early in 1970, with all markers in place and numbered, and with a guidebook ready, the Everglades Wilderness Waterway, a continuous path from Everglades City to Flamingo, officially opened.

Since that time, countless boaters and paddlers have carried that vintage guidebook or its 1985 edition on their Waterway trips.

TRIP PREPARATION

Much of the following information is pertinent for any and all paddling in Everglades National Park. It applies to all the routes in this book—those for thru-paddling the 99-mile Waterway and for the day and overnight routes described in Parts Two and Three. However, as the main focus of our guide is to lead you on a thru-paddle, we have anchored the elements of trip planning and preparation here.

CAMPING ON WATER, LAND, & SHORE

As noted in the Introduction, you must make reservations to use any of the camping facilities provided by the National Park Service (NPS). (Also see "Planning, Reservations, & Permits," on page 34.) Below, we elaborate on the three choices we touched on in the Introduction.

Chickees

Named after Native American Calusa and Seminole village structures, chickees are wooden platforms constructed on pilings to stand over the water. The standard-size chickee is 10 by 12 feet, so be sure to know your tent's dimensions before you plan to pitch it on one of these shelters. Also, hammering nails or screwing hooks into chickee boards is not permitted, so a freestanding tent is a necessity.

Open-sided with a roof and with a boardwalk leading to a privy, some chickees have ladders attached to the side. Some are single, and others are double (two platforms connected by a boardwalk), allowing more than one party to camp at the same site. Because they are positioned out on the water, chickees are often less buggy than ground sites. Chickee boards are hard, so you need a sleeping pad to ensure a comfortable night's sleep.

A word of caution: In areas with strong tidal fluctuations, a chickee whose platform is easily accessible at high tide might be out of reach at low tide. It is important to leave enough rope when you tie up at night so that if the tide falls, your boat isn't left hanging in the air on too-short ropes.

Ground Sites

These mall, cleared areas on old Calusa shell mounds are sites of Seminole and pioneer settlement. The Watson Place and Darwin's Place, for example, are locations where settlers in the Everglades eked out their living farming the land and trapping and fishing, many of them raising families. Ground sites have picnic tables and portable toilets, and some have docks. An advantage to a ground site is that you have easy access to your boat; disadvantages are that ground sites can be buggy because of the close vegetation, and raccoons can more easily reach your food and water supplies.

Beach Sites

Just as their name suggests, these campsites anchor you directly on the sandy shores of the Gulf of Mexico. Advantages are that you can swim, and you will have sea breezes and sunset views of the Gulf. If you are lucky, you might even see the green flash, that last green spark of light from the setting sun that can sometimes be seen on a clear evening. Disadvantages to beach sites are that raccoons can be a problem, but with food and water supplies well secured, we have never experienced difficulty beyond being awakened as raccoons attempted unsuccessfully to get into containers.

PLANNING, RESERVATIONS, & PERMITS

For use along with this guidebook, we urge you to get the free *Wilderness Trip Planner* from Everglades National Park by calling (305) 242-7700, or find it online at the park website, **nps.gov/ever.** (See "Navigation," on page 36, for information on additional maps and charts you should carry.)

Reservations are mandatory for camping along the Everglades Wilderness Waterway. You must make them *in person* at the Gulf Coast Visitor Center in Everglades City or the Flamingo Visitor Center within the 24-hour period prior to launch. Be aware that some older editions of the park's *Wilderness Trip Planner* indicate *incorrectly* that reservations could be made only "up to" 24 hours before launch, and this error has been replicated in some guidebooks.

The *Planner* also alerts you that in summertime, due to insect conditions, few people thru-paddle the Waterway, and the permit-writing desks may not be staffed. In such cases, you must follow self-registration instructions at the Flamingo or Gulf Coast Visitor Centers. But you *must* register. At press time, there is a $10 fee for a camping permit, plus $2 per person per day.

ITINERARIES

With cooler days and fewer mosquitoes, November–April is the most popular time for paddling the Waterway. Also, this is the dry season, when hurricanes and afternoon thunderstorms are not as much of a concern. The week between Christmas and New Year's Day is very busy, as are Presidents' Day weekend in February and spring break in March.

For the full Waterway trip, we recommend avoiding the summer months. The relentless mosquitoes, along with the chance of daily afternoon thunderstorms, could make paddling uncomfortable and dangerous. If you decide to take this on, please read very carefully Part Four, Summer Paddling, on page 201.

The Waterway can be paddled in 7–10 days. Your first decision will be whether to paddle north to south, or south to north. Create your itinerary, identifying your intended campsites before you go into the visitor center to make reservations. It's likely, however, that some of your chosen campsites will already be reserved. If this occurs, the park staff is helpful in choosing alternative campsites, but it's good to have substitutes already in mind. In high season, getting to the visitor center early may give you an advantage in securing your first choice of campsites. Starting mid-week might also improve your chances. Remember, however, that a second choice can often turn out to be better than the first. The first time we paddled the Waterway, we hadn't intended to go to Highland Beach; it turned out to be a highlight of the trip.

However you construct an itinerary, just be sure that you consider your paddling experience, your tested capability, and the fact that the distances between campsites can be considerable. Pay particular attention to reservations around The Nightmare (between the Broad River and the Harney River). You must paddle this section on a rising or high tide, or you risk getting stuck.

Once the journey is under way, the only reason to stay at campsites you have not reserved is in case of an emergency. As the park staff says, being tired is not an emergency. Be aware, also, that you will paddle farther than the 99 miles of the marked Waterway because many campsites and chickees lie a few hundred yards to a few miles from the marked channel.

You will need to shuttle back to your car when you finish your Waterway trip at Flamingo (if you travel north to south), or at Everglades City (if you travel south to north). We each have a carrier on top of our cars and sets of tie-downs. We leave one vehicle at one end of the Waterway and drive the other car with the canoe 130 miles to our launch at the other end. Some outfitters offer shuttle service for a fee (see Appendix 2, Launch Sites, on page 269, and Appendix 4, Resource Overview, on page 278). Or you might ask a friend to shuttle you. There is no charge to leave your car for the week at either the Flamingo or the Everglades City visitor center.

NAVIGATION

Although we include GPS markings in this guidebook, we prefer the adventure and challenge of navigating with map and compass, paying attention to positions of sun and moon, light and shadow, feeling a closer relationship with the wilderness through which we move. This is a matter of preference for each paddler. You will decide what is right for you, but if you do choose GPS, be sure to take the appropriate NOAA (National Oceanic and Atmospheric Administration) chart or Waterproof Chart and a compass as a backup. Technology can fail and batteries die.

In constructing the north-to-south and south-to-north routes in this book, we have tried to be clear and detailed in our instructions. However, these paddling areas are complex, and you will be weaving among myriad mangrove islands. Often you cannot see from one Wilderness Waterway marker to the next, and sometimes there are miles between markers. In addition, *some markers may be missing.* Please do not rely on this guide alone or on free park maps and brochures or even the more detailed National Geographic Everglades Topo map for navigation. You will need navigational charts. We carry both NOAA and Waterproof charts (see below), and we enjoy having a set of maps for each paddler. This facilitates consultation when the navigation gets tricky.

- NOAA navigational charts 11430, 11432, and 11433 collectively cover the extent of the Waterway. Call NOAA at (301) 436-6990, or visit **nauticalcharts.noaa.gov.**
- Waterproof Charts 39 and 41 also cover the Wilderness Waterway and can be ordered from Waterproof Charts, Inc. Call (800) 423-9026, or visit **waterproofcharts.com.**

These charts are also for sale at local marinas and other outlets (see Appendix 3, Outfitters, Suppliers, & Canoe/Kayak Rentals, on page 275). Each type of map has its advantages. Waterproof Charts are, as the name suggests, waterproof. The NOAA charts are paper, making it easy to mark your compass headings right on the map. The Waterproof Charts mark the GPS coordinates for campsites. NOAA charts do not.

Protect your charts in transparent, large, waterproof map cases, available from outdoor-supply stores.

In addition, you must have a compass. We recommend a canoe/kayak compass that you can attach to your boat for monitoring your direction during travel, as well as a handheld compass, the kind with the rotating dial, to plot compass headings if that becomes necessary.

Following a course while crossing bays can be tricky, especially since different mangrove shorelines look similar at a distance and openings between islands are usually not visible until you are near them. While paddling the Waterway, you will learn navigation tricks just by careful observation. For example, watch for powerboaters going in or out of otherwise invisible passages, and look for lighter-against-darker shades of the mangrove shorelines, which may indicate the channel you are seeking. A pair of binoculars will help you spot distant markers.

SAFETY

Never forget that you are embarking on a wilderness adventure. Paddling the full Wilderness Waterway is not for beginners. Although you are sometimes in sheltered creeks, the majority of the trip is through open bays, where winds regularly reach 15 knots (more than 17 mph), and higher winds are not unusual. Do not take chances. Below are some critical pointers:

- Check the long-range weather conditions before you embark. Once you are a few days out on the Waterway (or on the long day paddles or overnight paddles in Parts Two and Three of this guide), it will be difficult to turn back if conditions suddenly worsen as a front comes through.
- If the wind is strong, hug the shore and take rest breaks on the leeward side of islands. You may need to tack to get across a bay to prevent waves from hitting you broadside. Turn the bow of your boat into the wake left by speeding motorboaters.
- Wear your spray skirt when kayaking, and bungee down a tarp to cover your gear if you are in a canoe.
- Wear your personal flotation device (PFD). We recommend those specifically designed for use while paddling. For lightweight comfort, you might consider the suspender type with a CO2 cartridge and pull cord for inflation. Women may note that some modern PFD designs are specifically tailored for a woman's shape.
- Keep a whistle on a cord attached to your PFD, and remember the U.S. Coast Guard (USCG) boating regulations: five short blasts is the danger signal.
- Pack flares for emergencies.

Tide Charts

Carry a tide chart for the area and the days when you will be out. Tide charts are available at both of the visitor centers, or you can download charts (which we have found easier to read) at **saltwatertides.com.** We have found their usefulness to be limited, however, in the inland channels where tides may vary from those listed for the Gulf. In most cases, by remaining attentive, you can figure out how the tides are moving and when they are likely to change. Although awareness of tides is more important in some areas than in others, it is obviously easier to paddle with a tide than against one, and all areas of the Waterway are under some tidal influence. Tidal awareness is particularly important when you are tackling The Nightmare route, as a low tide can leave you stranded for quite a while.

Communication

Depending upon the time of year, you may encounter many other people on your trip, or you may spend days without seeing another soul. You will not have cell phone service along most of the Waterway. To get weather reports, carry a waterproof handheld marine radio, which has a 5-mile range. The marine radio's channel 16 provides access to the USCG emergency channel. You might consider purchasing or borrowing a satellite phone or a personal locator beacon (PLB), a safety device that "spots" your location in emergencies.

As soon as you have made your campsite reservations, contact a friend and share your float plan and expected arrival date. Give your friend the park emergency number, (305) 242-7740, in case you do not arrive by the designated date. Be responsible in keeping to your timetable, but never paddle into known danger just to arrive on time.

Lost?

If you become totally lost, follow the falling tide west to the Gulf. Once there, paddle north along the coastline until you get the attention of another boater or until you find a marked channel or another landmark (such as a marked NPS campsite). These markers will help you determine where you are on your navigation charts.

Weather Precautions

If you are paddling during the dry season, the likelihood of thunderstorms is low, but they can occur. If you are on the water and you hear thunder, paddle into a little side stream in the mangroves or hug the shore. Wear your PFD, and be sure to wait a half hour after a lightning storm before going back into open water. Consider taking a cardiopulmonary resuscitation (CPR) course before your trip; in case lightning strikes, a stunned victim can be resuscitated. You can't call 911 when you are on the Waterway, although a marine radio is helpful in emergency situations. For considerably more information about thunderstorms, see Part Four, Summer Paddling, on page 201.

To Your Health

Heatstroke and hypothermia are life-threatening. To prevent heatstroke, drink plenty of fluids and do not paddle to the point of exhaustion in direct sun. Wear a hat and take breaks to cool off in the shade at the side of the Waterway. Splash some water on yourself to cool down. The opposite extreme is hypothermia, a dangerous lowering of one's body temperature. Hypothermia can be a risk in the winter season or when cold fronts come through in the fall and spring. To prevent hypothermia, stay dry and warm, and be alert to signs of hypothermia in your companions, such as shivering, poor coordination, and confusion. Take measures immediately to dry and warm up the victim.

Monitor your companions to be sure that they aren't stressed by either the cold or the heat. People often do not recognize their own symptoms.

Sunburn can be painful and dangerous, so remember to stop paddling often to apply sunscreen and lip balm. Drink plenty of water to avoid dehydration. Drink regularly. Don't wait until you're thirsty. When you're thirsty, you are already becoming dehydrated.

Critters

Regarding snakes and alligators—to expand for a moment on what we have already said in the Introduction (see pages 14–15)—you probably won't see a single snake, even on the full Waterway paddling expedition. They are shy and want as little to do with you as you do with them. But always use normal caution when exploring tall grass or walking around ground sites.

On a thru-paddle up or down the Waterway, you will see alligators and occasionally the endangered American crocodile. As noted previously, they will slip into the water if you paddle close to them sunning on the banks. But remember, never dump leftover food into the water, and watch for these reptiles as you near chickees and ground sites because previous campers may not have been as cautious as they should have been.

See page 11 for a reminder about the problems of insects and page 14 for a refresher on the dangers of oysters.

SANITATION

Do not assume that you can paddle to the shore, step out, and relieve yourself. The only sandy shores are on the Gulf; the rest of the Waterway is lined with interlacing mangrove roots, muck, or oyster beds. The Wilderness is not the place to be shy. You will need to urinate directly into the water. With a little finesse, both men and women can manage to do this.

The following suggestion works well for women in a canoe: paddle over to the mangroves and, while your paddling partner leans the opposite direction to steady the boat, turn sideways and hang your backside over the side of the canoe. Kayakers will need a different approach. Shelley Johnson, in her section "To Pee or Not to Pee" in *Sea Kayaking: A Woman's Guide,* writes of a friend who "cuts the top of a dishwashing soap container at a handy angle" to funnel urine into a jar to pour over the edge. A similar device, called a Freshette, can be ordered from Campmor; visit **campmor.com.**

At campsites, use the portable toilets, which come equipped with toilet paper. Bring one roll just in case and for use on Highland Beach. If there is no portable toilet, make your cathole far from the campsite, back in the brush. Bring a hand trowel, dig a 6-inch hole, and bury your solid waste and toilet paper, or pack the paper out. Take your head net (see "Clothing," on page 44) when you go into the woods, because once in the shade you will encounter mosquitoes.

There are few beaches, and there are alligators *in* the Waterway, so do not anticipate taking a bath during your trip. Premoistened towelettes are handy, but do not deposit them into the privy. Be sure to pack them out. If you bring sanitary supplies, pack them out too.

PADDLING GEAR

We use a canoe on our Wilderness Waterway trips, although many people travel in kayaks. You can rent both in the Everglades. (See

Appendix 3, Outfitters, Suppliers, & Canoe/Kayak Rentals, on page 275.) Rentals often do not have adequate rope for tying up, so when renting, be sure to bring extra rope.

If you're canoeing, bring spare paddles tied to the struts so they don't float away if your boat tips. Carry a water pump and a large marine sponge for bailing; a cut-off plastic jug also works just fine. To keep the waves or rain from splashing into your canoe, cover your entire load with a tarp secured with bungee cords stretched across the gunwales. Kayakers need a spray skirt and paddle tether.

We sometimes use foldable seats for back support as we paddle, and we find them useful for sitting in the tent or on the chickee at the end of the day. If you have space, you might bring small collapsible camp chairs for even more comfort at your campsite.

Be sure to have long ropes tied to each end of the boat to secure it to the chickee at night. Remember that the tide differential can be extreme on some of the chickees, so once you unload, keep a lot of slack in the ropes. Kayakers often bring their boats up onto the chickee at night.

To keep your canoe from floating away if you capsize, carry a small anchor attached by a 15-foot rope, and be sure it isn't buried under your gear, where it will be of no use to you if your boat tips. Lay it on top so it will fall quickly to the bottom in the event of capsizing.

If you paddle at night, bow and stern lights are mandatory. A long-beam flashlight can be helpful when searching for markers at night.

Dry bags are essential for keeping clothing and supplies from getting wet. Using different colors for different types of supplies can be helpful—or use clear ones so you can determine contents at a glance.

CAMPING SUPPLIES

You will need a freestanding tent. Primarily this is for protection from mosquitoes, but it also provides shelter from rain on the nights that you do not stay on a chickee, and at times when the wind might blow rain under the chickee roof.

If conditions are windy, you should set up your tent immediately and stow your gear inside. That will anchor the tent on the chickee and will keep your lighter gear from flying away. At times the wind may blow so hard that you will want to secure your tent to the chickee posts with bungees or ropes.

Weather can vary, no matter the season. Unless you paddle in the middle of summer, you may have a warm evening followed by a chilly night. So bring a sleeping bag. You will appreciate being in the bag on cooler nights, and you can sleep on top of the bag if the weather is warm.

To assure some comfort in the wilderness, don't forget these items: a sleeping pad, a camp pillow, and a headlamp to read and write by at night and for finding your way to the privy in the dark. Consider bringing a headlamp with a red-light feature that helps you keep your night vision. Be sure to pack spare lithium batteries, which, reportedly, last up to three times longer than regular batteries.

CLOTHING

Because of the intense sun, a hat with a brim is a necessity. Any hat that shades your eyes is fine, but your neck needs protection too. Many fishermen wear hats with a long bill in front and a flap to cover the back of the neck.

Bring a lightweight waterproof jacket to wear in case it rains. A jacket is preferable to a poncho, which can flap in the wind. Because you don't want to hunt for your rain jacket when a squall develops, keep your raingear within easy reach in the top of a dry bag. Bring a fleece jacket for cool evenings and mornings. Fleece sheds water and is cozy. Keep your fleece handy at the top of a dry bag in case a chilly wind picks up while you paddle.

Take at least one pair of lightweight long pants for protection from the sun in the daytime and from mosquitoes and the chill in the evenings. We suggest at least one long-sleeved shirt for sun protection during the day and for mosquito protection in the evening and early morning. Cotton is cool but does not wick moisture. If it gets wet, it stays wet the whole trip. We recommend nylon or another quick-drying fabric, and many are impregnated with sunblock and mosquito repellent that lasts for dozens of washings; you can rinse out dirty clothes and bungee them on the boat to dry during the day. If you are paddling in the winter, pack a pair of polypropylene long underwear. Bring socks for buggy or chilly nights. Additional reminders:

- Wear water shoes or sneakers. If you step into the water, you must wear protective shoes because of the sharp oyster shells.
- Pack a head net to protect yourself from mosquitoes. You may never wear it, but it takes almost no space, and if you need it, you'll be happy to have it.
- Wear paddling gloves. Lightweight, all-purpose exercise gloves will serve the purpose. Gloves protect your hands from blisters and prevent sunburn.
- Don't forget to pack bandannas. They dry quickly and serve many purposes—pot holder, headband, tissue, washcloth, or towel.

As food for thought, a kayak racer once stopped by briefly to chat when we were camping at Plate Creek Chickee and advised us to have a separate dry set of clothes saved for emergency situations.

COOKING SUPPLIES

Nothing that produces ash (including wood or charcoal fires) may be used on ground sites or on chickees. Campfires are permitted only on beach sites. So be sure to bring a campstove. We use one, or sometimes two, single-burner propane stoves; the stove element screws directly onto the top of the propane cartridge. We generally bring four full propane cartridges for two people. The propane required will vary according to what you cook and wind conditions. If you like to dine well out there, it is no fun to contemplate eating cold food toward the end of your trip. Worse yet not to have coffee on your final days. Don't forget at least two butane lighters. They can be cranky, and sometimes when one won't work, the other will. Always have a box of matches in a waterproof container, just in case.

If your vehicle is a kayak, you will need cooking equipment that's very compact. You can get fuel canisters and a burner made specifically to fit through your hatches.

Making coffee

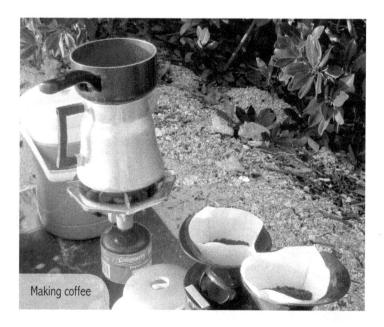

We use one cook kit with nested pots (the lids of which become frying pans) and a stirring spoon, paring knife, and spatula. Each of us uses a wide, shallow Corelle bowl, which serves well as both bowl and plate; each has a knife, fork, and spoon, and a thermal cup for coffee or tea.

Be aware that chickee boards are spaced far apart. We expect that many a knife, fork, and spoon have fallen between the boards over the years, and we confess that we contributed a spoon of our own. To prevent dropping things between the boards, we've learned to spread out a tarp before cooking. To wash your dishes, bring a scrubbie.

We like good coffee, and we use a Melita one-cup drip device to brew a cup at a time. (A funnel works just as well.) If you're a coffee lover, bring filters and plenty of good ground java.

FOOD

Take care with the food you pack. A good cup of coffee at the start of the day, a granola bar after a hard stretch of paddling, a bowl of hot soup after setting up your tent in the evening, and a fine dinner can be rewards for hard work on the Waterway. The definition of good food is a very personal matter, however. For some, the best camp cooking is the quickest, easiest thing that will get calories into the stomach: open a can of beans and a loaf of bread and you're happy. For others (we fall into this category), at the end of a day of hard paddling, you want something special, so here are some tips for the Waterway gourmet.

Snacks

Snacks matter. We burn a lot of energy out there, so we try to routinely have snacks midmorning and midafternoon, and occasionally another one along the way. Sometimes we rely almost entirely on granola bars and fruit-and-nut bars. Sometimes we've had cheese sticks and crackers or Babybel cheese with biscotti. Sometimes almonds and fresh fruit, either apples or oranges. Whatever you decide upon, don't leave snacks to chance. Plan them as carefully as you plan meals. Pack them in a separate container, apart from other foodstuffs, and be sure that you can get to them easily when you need them. We stash ours under the canoe seats.

Breakfast

We've learned to make breakfast easy: coffee and oatmeal with walnuts and fruit. By varying the fruit, we have a sense of not having exactly the same thing every day. The only cooking that has to be done is to boil water. We use the water for making good, strong coffee and for pouring into our bowls waiting with oatmeal and raisins, nuts, dried fruit, or fresh blueberries. Our blueberries have stayed good for almost a week. For oatmeal, we use a mixture of about three-fourths quick oats and, for texture, about one-fourth old-fashioned oats. We measure carefully in advance to be sure that we will have the right number of servings (plus some extra just in case) and put all of the oats, along with a scoop, into a plastic container with a tightly fitting lid. We sprinkle the oats and fruit with a little dried milk before pouring on the hot water.

Lunch

We keep lunch simple too. Peanut butter sandwiches. No jelly. Just peanut butter. Following peanut butter sandwiches, we usually have fresh fruit and sometimes mint patties from the cooler. Occasionally we have tuna sandwiches made with seasoned tuna from a foil packet that needs no refrigeration. Whatever you choose for lunch fare, when you've been out there awhile, working hard, it's great to tie up to a marker or a mangrove, stretch your legs out over the load, and enjoy grand, simple fare.

Dinner & Recipes

Ah, dinner! Now, for us, that's another category of food altogether. The paragraphs below explain how canoeists can have delicious meals throughout the Waterway trip. Kayakers will need to have more of a backpacking mentality because of the limited space, but it is still possible to create savory meals with pasta, spices, foil-packaged tuna and chicken, fresh fruit, and vegetables. If you have the time and ambition, you can freeze-dry meals. Just be sure to bring more than you think you will need. Paddling all day will make you hungry.

For us, a favorite meal for the first night out is Cuban pork chops with black beans, a recipe we are happy to share here. This can be prepared well in advance and frozen. Many dishes lend themselves to a paddling journey—just start out with a pre-chilled cooler and be sure the food itself is frozen.

CUBAN PORK CHOPS

8 thin pork chops
salt
pepper
¼ teaspoon ground cumin
¼ teaspoon dried oregano
3–5 garlic cloves, crushed
¼ cup orange juice
⅛ cup fresh lime juice
⅛ cup fresh lemon juice
(If fresh sour oranges are available, use ½ cup of sour-orange juice instead of the orange, lime, and lemon juices.)
2 large onions, thinly sliced
3 tablespoons olive oil
½ cup dry sherry

At least a day or two before your departure—to allow time for freezing the cooked meat—rub the chops with salt and pepper, then with a paste you make of the cumin, oregano, and garlic. Place the chops in a glass bowl and add the juices (or sour-orange juice) and thinly sliced onions. Marinate in the refrigerator 3–4 hours.

Remove chops from the marinade, reserving the marinade. Pat the chops dry with paper towels. Heat the oil in a sauté pan, and quickly brown the chops on both sides. Add the reserved marinade and the sherry.

Reduce the heat, cover, and cook 18–22 minutes, until chops are tender. When cooled, place the chops and the cooked onions in plastic freezer bags, apportioning according to the servings you will need on the Waterway, and freeze until time to pack for travel.

Waterway Black Beans

½ medium onion, chopped
2 garlic cloves, chopped
1 green bell pepper, chopped
¼ cup olive oil
1 large tomato, chopped
2 (16-ounce) cans black beans
Several dashes Tabasco sauce
1 tablespoon red wine vinegar
1 teaspoon ground cumin
Salt and pepper
½ cup broth or water

Cook onion, garlic, and bell pepper in the oil, over low heat, about 10 minutes, stirring often. Add the chopped tomato and cook another 5–7 minutes. Add beans (do not drain or rinse them), Tabasco, vinegar, cumin, salt and pepper to taste, and broth or water, stirring. Cover and simmer about 15–20 minutes. Cool. Spoon into plastic bags for freezing, apportioning according to how much you will need for one or two meals.

Food Freshness & Safety The night before departure, fill the cooler with ice so that it will be cold when you put food into it. Everything you put into the cooler should be cold or frozen so that nothing will immediately begin to bring down the temperature. The ice that was used for pre-chilling will be discarded, replaced with whatever you intend to use to keep the chill—blue ices, dry ice, or (our favorite) a large chunk of ice that you have pre-frozen in a half-gallon or gallon container. A large ice block will last longer and prolong chilling more effectively than ice cubes or crushed ice. Starting out this way, you can plan to have whatever you would like for dinner the first three nights out—either food prepared and frozen in advance or the materials that you will need for constructing the meal on-site.

After the third night, you can continue to have fresh vegetables. An avocado that's hard when you set out will generally be perfect by the fourth night. Cauliflower florets, Brussels sprouts, and red and green peppers easily keep a week or longer, as will tomatoes if they are not too ripe when you set out. Potatoes, onions, and carrots are fine for 10 days or longer. Generally, if you select vegetables carefully, they hold up well. When you're halfway through the trip and the cooler is no longer cool, just be sure to keep your veggies dry so they won't mold.

With our veggies, we enjoy pasta concoctions, couscous, Stove Top stuffing, and rice. We no longer cook regular rice or brown rice from scratch, however, because it takes a long time and uses a lot of cooking fuel. We've found some quick rice mixes, including a wild rice mix, that we like well enough.

For seafood or meat, foil packets available in most supermarkets have been great: favorites include seasoned tuna, salmon, chicken chunks, and crab (we've made great crab cakes, improvising from the recipe on the packet). The packets take a minimum of space and are much lighter in weight than cans, giving us little to pack out.

We like to have soup several times on the trip, especially on chilly evenings. Soup is good as a main course and sometimes as a first course at dinnertime. Again, we avoid cans, taking instead boxed soups, for lighter packaging and easy packing out.

We bring and use the small touches that enhance the food—lemon or lime, cumin, bay leaf, thyme, salt, and fresh pepper.

We plan very carefully with established written menus for each night. Once we're out there, we often vary these, but it's a way of being sure that we will have sufficient supplies without hauling a lot more than we need. We have learned, however, that it is important to carry food for at least one more day than we anticipate being out. We've never been stranded without supplies, but once we came sufficiently close that we have become attentive to the possibility. We pack now for a day and a half beyond our anticipated trip time. Just in case.

WATER

You will have to carry your entire freshwater supply:

- There are no sources of freshwater along the 99-mile Waterway.
- The water in this part of the Everglades is too brackish to filter and drink (though, in a pinch, you can consider cooking with brackish water).
- Standard recommendations note that you should carry 1 gallon of water per person per day.

For a canoe, you can handle your water supply several different ways, but don't head out with a bunch of loose plastic gallon jugs that raccoons can chew into. Use hard-sided water containers, 3–5 gallons each. Some people use 5-gallon Home Depot containers with snap-on lids. If you want the convenience of gallon jugs, you can put several jugs into hard-sided boxes and bungee the boxes tightly. We have done this, and although raccoons tried to get into the jugs, they didn't succeed. Kayakers can buy specially designed water bags to tuck in their boats.

While 1 gallon of water per person per day is recommended, a little extra won't hurt if you have room. You may not use all the water you bring, but we have learned that the weight of the water serves as good ballast on windy, wavy days.

One more note about water: Continuous hydration is important. Each paddler should carry a water bottle within easy reach in the boat. In a canoe, a water bottle holder that is attached to the seat with Velcro will make it easy for you to drink often. For kayakers, a hydration pack might be just the thing.

THRU-PADDLING THE EVERGLADES WILDERNESS WATERWAY

In this book, we have organized maps and text into 21 sections to cover the 99-mile Wilderness Waterway route. From north to south, the sections are *numbered* 1 to 21; from south to north, they are *alphabetized* A to U.

You may paddle the Waterway section by section in either direction. But to avoid duplicate maps, we have labeled each map by number/letter. You may use this book from pages 57–115 for the north-to-south route; and backwards, from pages 115–57, for the south-to-north route.

For example, note that Section 1/U, below, *begins* section 1 of the north-to-south route, in Everglades City. Conversely, the same map and somewhat varied text also represents section U, which *completes* the south-to-north paddle, in Everglades City. See the charts on the next pages for a quick reference to all the sections, in both directions, and for each section's page number.

In addition to the 21 sections we describe in detail in this book, The Historical Route is another passage along part of the Wilderness Waterway. However, because this route crosses Whitewater Bay, it can be quite hazardous for paddlers and we do not recommend it. For more information, see Map 22 and brief text, on page 115.

North-to-south Thru-paddle Route: SECTIONS 1–21

South-to-north Thru-paddle Route: SECTIONS A–U

Whether you are heading north or south, you can expect to observe certain landmarks, flora, and fauna within each section that you paddle. We provide detailed descriptions primarily in the north-to-south text, but we include additional information—or the reverse perspective if pertinent—in the accompanying text for each section of the south-to-north route.

MARKERS

The historical Wilderness Waterway ran from marker 1 through marker 130, south to north. Currently there is no Wilderness Waterway marker 1 at Flamingo, and there are no markers 128, 129, or 130 in the Everglades City area.

Thus, currently, the Wilderness Waterway markers run from number 2, near Flamingo, to marker 127 at Chokoloskee Bay. As a general rule, even-numbered markers are to your left and odd-numbered markers are to your right as you travel north to south (from Everglades City to Flamingo) and even-numbered markers are to the right and odd-numbered markers to the left as you travel south to north (Flamingo to Everglades City). Wilderness Waterway markers are brown arrow shapes with white numbers. They are positioned on poles out in the water or near the shore. You will also see—and our route directions also reference—USCG markers; they are red triangles or green squares. *The maps in this guide show triangles for Waterway markers and circles for USCG markers.*

As you paddle, you will find that weather and time may have caused some Waterway markers to disappear. However, you can be certain that the NPS works hard to maintain these markers. Make note of missing markers and report them at the end of your trip. Use your map and compass skills to confirm your position if markers are missing.

Appendix 7, on page 288, provides a handy list of the GPS coordinates for all Wilderness Waterway markers and campsites.

(We also include relevant GPS coordinates in the introduction to each route description.)

SECTION 1/U:

EVERGLADES CITY (GULF COAST VISITOR CENTER)/ CHOKOLOSKEE ISLAND (SOUTH END)

Gulf Coast Visitor Center: N25° 50.730' W81° 23.234'
Chokoloskee Island: N25° 48.537' W81° 21.442'
Estimated paddling distance: 3.5 miles

NORTH TO SOUTH:
Everglades City to Chokoloskee Island

Launch your canoe or kayak to the right of the Gulf Coast Visitor Center at Everglades National Park. The park provides a wheelbarrow to carry your gear from your car to the launch site on Chokoloskee Bay. Make every effort to launch near high tide because launching at low tide may necessitate pulling your craft through thigh-deep mud before you can climb into your boat and paddle off. (For alternative, fee-based launch sites, see Appendix 2, Launch Sites, on page 269.)

Just before you reach the bridge, you have two choices—the Causeway Canal route or the Chokoloskee Bay route.

Be aware that launching on an outgoing tide will make it difficult to paddle under the bridge if you are planning to take the Causeway Canal route. On the other hand, the advantage of the Causeway Canal route is that you avoid the waves and oyster beds of Chokoloskee Bay. For the canal route, turn left (east) and paddle under the causeway bridge and then turn right, heading southeast along the canal that follows the eastern side of the Chokoloskee Causeway. Be sure to stay to the far left (east) as you paddle the canal because the western (right) side can become too shallow to paddle.

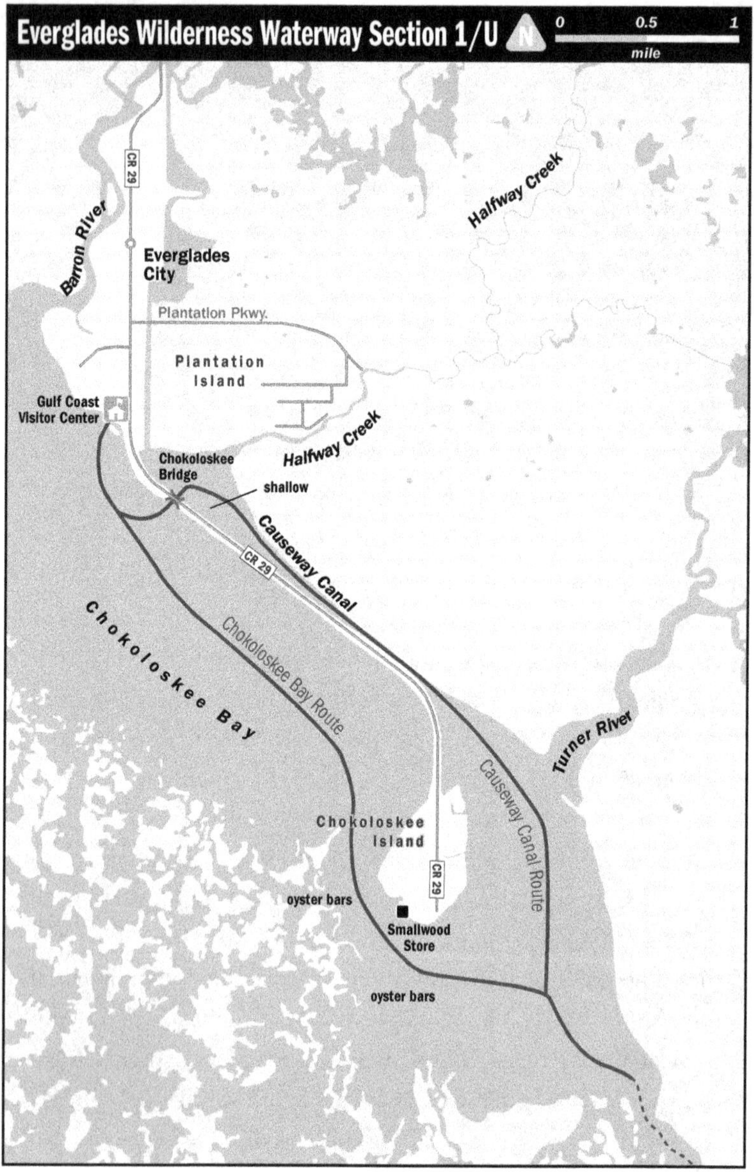
Everglades Wilderness Waterway Section 1/U
N
0
0.5
1
mile
CR 29
Barron River
Everglades City
Halfway Creek
Plantation Pkwy.
Plantation Island
Gulf Coast Visitor Center
Halfway Creek
Chokoloskee Bridge
shallow
Causeway Canal
CR 29
Chokoloskee Bay
Chokoloskee Bay Route
Turner River
Causeway Canal Route
Chokoloskee Island
CR 29
oyster bars
Smallwood Store
oyster bars

The advantage of the Chokoloskee Bay route is that it conveniently passes Historic Smallwood Store (see page 260), and it makes a delightful place to stop for a break. If the tide is ripping out under the bridge and you find that you cannot paddle against the tide, take this route for sure. On the Chokoloskee Bay route, continue southeast down the bay and pass Chokoloskee Island on your left (east). Watch out for the oyster beds.

SOUTH TO NORTH:
Chokoloskee Island to Everglades City

Heading for your takeout by way of the Causeway Canal route, pass Chokoloskee Island to your left (west) and the Turner River to your right (east). (See "Chokoloskee Island" on page 248.) You

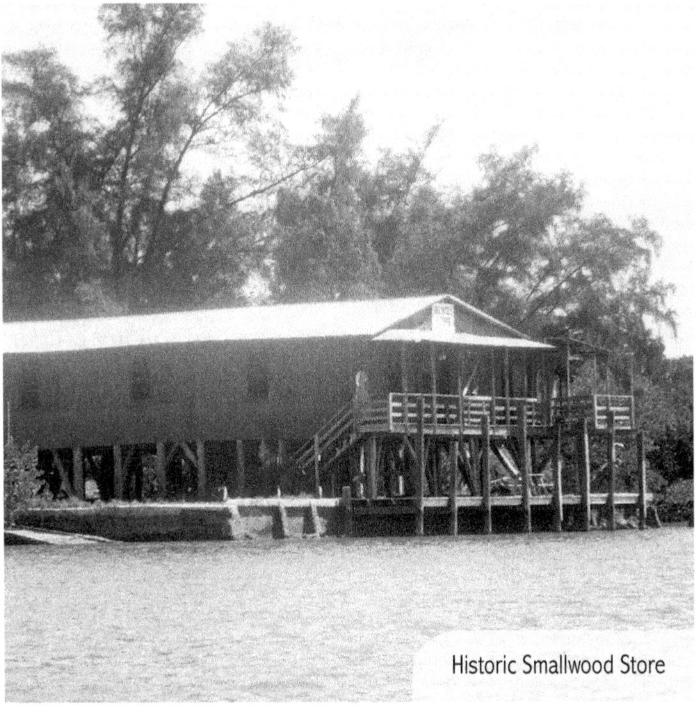

Historic Smallwood Store

will be funneled into the canal that lies to the right of the Chokoloskee Causeway. The advantage of this route is that the canal itself offers a calm passage with great birding. The disadvantage is that you may face a ripping incoming tide as you paddle under the bridge.

Stay to the right in this canal, as the left side can become impassable at low tide. When you come to the bridge, turn left. Pass under the bridge, turn right, and head to your takeout point at Gulf Coast Visitor Center, Everglades National Park, in Everglades City.

If you are coming in via the Chokoloskee Bay route, paddle northwest across the bay, passing Chokoloskee Island to your right (east). This route is often wavier than the canal option, and the shallow bay is lined with oyster beds. The advantage is that you will pass Historic Smallwood Store on the west side of Chokoloskee Island. Now a museum, the store is worth a visit, particularly if you are waiting for the tide to come up for your takeout at Everglades City. You can purchase your first cold drink since you left Flamingo.

Leaving Smallwood Store, paddle northwest from the northern end of the island, passing the Chokoloskee Bridge on your right. Gulf Coast Visitor Center will appear shortly on your right. The takeout point lies immediately past the visitor center.

Make every effort to take out near high tide because there is no dock. Low tide may necessitate dragging your boat through thigh-deep mud. The park provides a cart to carry your gear to your vehicle.

SECTION 2/T:

CHOKOLOSKEE ISLAND/LOPEZ RIVER CAMPSITE OR CROOKED CREEK CHICKEE

Chokoloskee Island: N25° 48.537' W81° 21.442'
Lopez River Campsite: N25° 47.275' W81° 18.374'
Crooked Creek Chickee: N25° 47.785' W81° 17.922'
Estimated paddling distance, Chokoloskee Island/Lopez River Campsite: 4 miles
Estimated paddling distance, Chokoloskee Island/Crooked Creek Chickee: 5 miles

NORTH TO SOUTH:
Chokoloskee Island to Lopez River Campsite or Crooked Creek Chickee

Passing Chokoloskee Island, paddle in a southeasterly direction down the bay to marker 127 and turn left (east) onto the Lopez River. Keep paddling in an easterly direction.

Motorboaters frequent this portion of the Waterway and, because this is not a no-wake zone, these boaters often travel fast; stay alert to the sound of motors.

Approximately 2 miles up the Lopez River, you will come to the Lopez River Campsite on your right with its old cistern and modern privy. If you are not staying here overnight, this is a good spot to have lunch in the shade and wander around the remains of Gregorio Lopez's old 1890s homesite (see page 230). You can understand why Lopez chose this fine spot on the river with its proximity to the Gulf of Mexico and to Chokoloskee. See if you can decipher the markings on the vault-shaped structures on the front of the cistern. If you are staying at Crooked Creek Chickee, continue northeast on the Lopez until it bends to the west. At this point, turn off the Lopez into Crooked Creek. This is the first stream branching off the Lopez to the

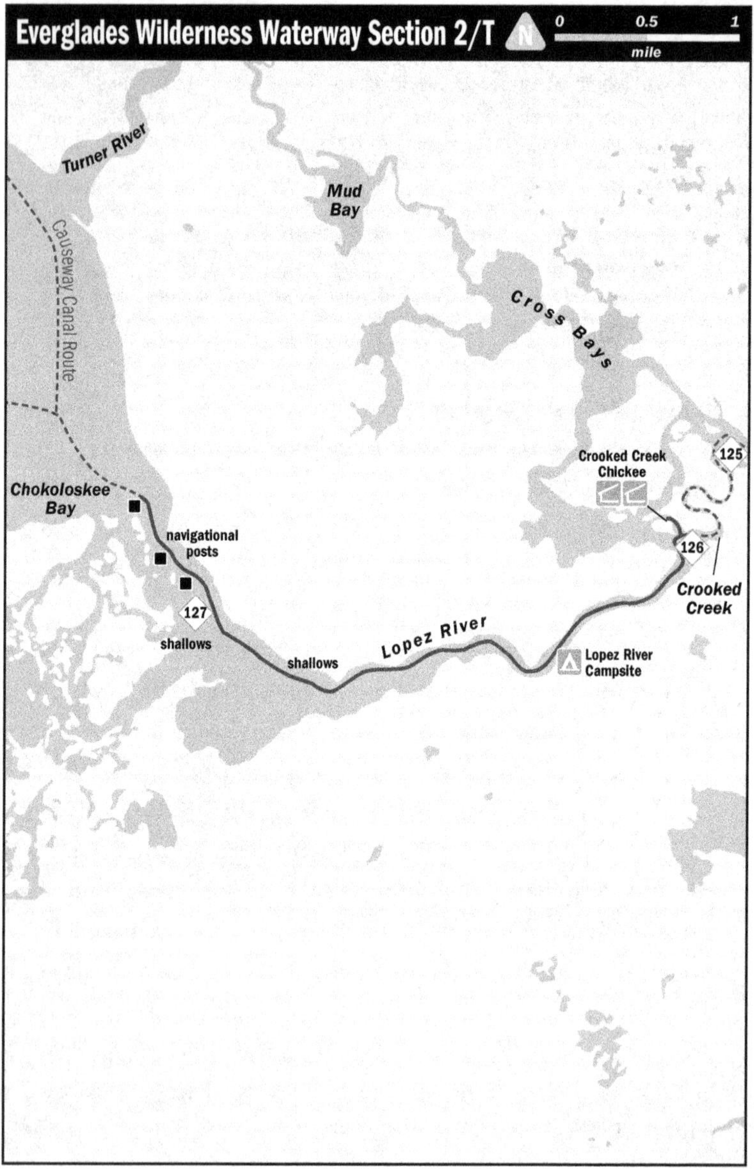
Everglades Wilderness Waterway Section 2/T
N
0
0.5
1
mile
Turner River
Mud Bay
Causeway Canal Route
Cross Bays
Crooked Creek Chickee
125
Chokoloskee Bay
navigational posts
126
Crooked Creek
127
shallows
shallows
Lopez River
Lopez River Campsite

right (east). As you turn, marker 126 will be on your right. The chickee is behind the mangrove island to your left.

SOUTH TO NORTH: Crooked Creek Chickee or Lopez River Campsite to Chokoloskee Island

From the Crooked Creek Chickee, return to the creek that shortly joins the Lopez River, and paddle southwest. Lopez River Campsite lies about 1 mile on the left. About 2 miles beyond the campsite, keep right through the bend, and you will enter Chokoloskee Bay at marker 127. Paddle northwest into Chokoloskee Bay, and determine which route you will take around the island to finish up your trip, either the Causeway Canal route or the Chokoloskee Bay route (see advantages and disadvantages in the north-to-south route description, above). You will likely see busy pelicans and cormorants fishing in the shallow bay.

SECTION 3/S

LOPEZ RIVER CAMPSITE OR CROOKED CREEK CHICKEE/MARKER 123

Lopez River Campsite: N25° 47.275' W81° 18.374'
Crooked Creek Chickee: N25° 47.785' W81° 17.922'
Marker 123: N25° 48.050' W81° 17.363'
Estimated paddling distance, Lopez River Campsite/marker 123: 2.5 miles
Estimated paddling distance, Crooked Creek Chickee/marker 123: 1.5 miles

NORTH TO SOUTH: Lopez River Campsite or Crooked Creek Chickee to Marker 123

Leaving the Lopez River Campsite, follow the river, looking for the first channel to the right (east) and marker 126. Here, where the river bends west, turn right into Crooked Creek. If you stayed at Crooked Creek Chickee, paddle back to the creek and turn left (east) to follow this serpentine channel. Continue along Crooked

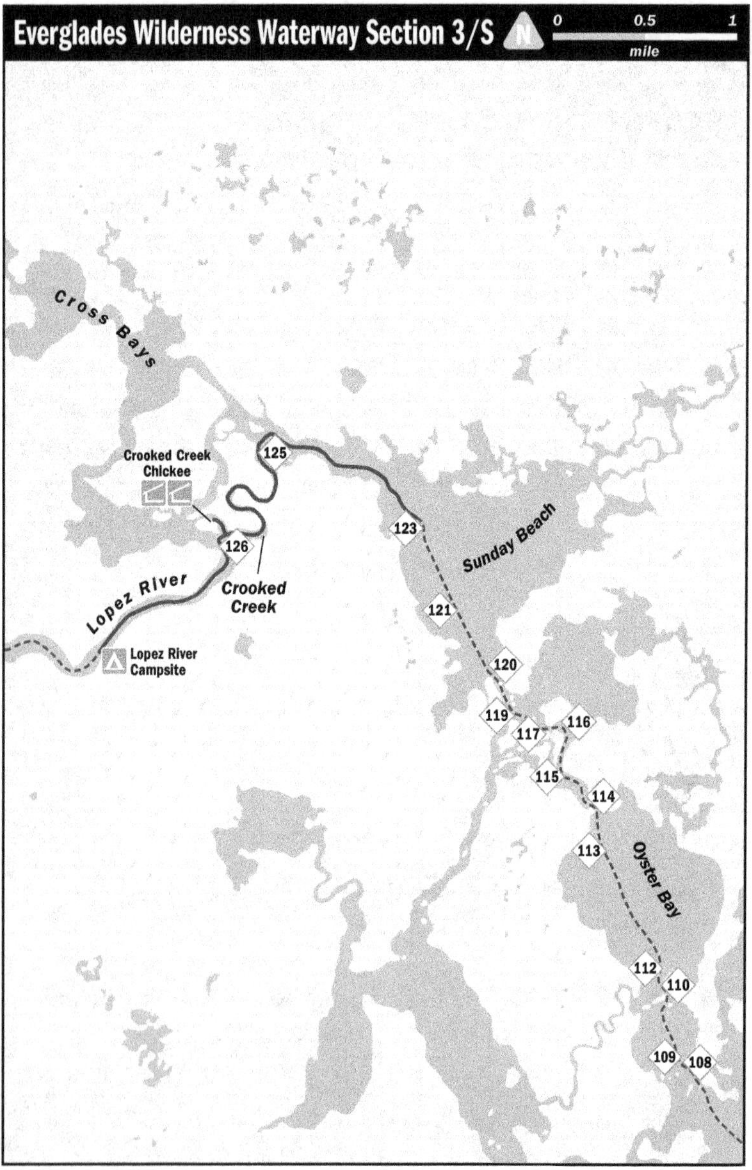
Everglades Wilderness Waterway Section 3/S
N
0
0.5
1
mile
Cross Bays
Crooked Creek
Chickee
125
123
126
Sunday Beach
Lopez River
Crooked
Creek
121
Lopez River
Campsite
120
119
116
117
115
114
113
Oyster Bay
112
110
109
108

Creek until it turns right (east) at marker 125 into Sunday Bay. Enter Sunday Bay and paddle south to marker 123.

SOUTH TO NORTH: Marker 123 to Crooked Creek Chickee or Lopez River Campsite

From marker 123, follow Sunday Bay as it curves northwest to marker 125, where you make a sharp left (south) into the serpentine channel called Crooked Creek. Follow this about 1 mile until you see the Lopez River. The Crooked Creek Chickee lies to your right behind the mangrove island at the mouth of Crooked Creek. If you plan to stay at the Lopez River Campsite, continue on Crooked Creek, which shortly intersects with the Lopez River. Turn left onto the Lopez and paddle about 1 mile downriver to the Lopez River Campsite on your left. This campsite is easy to spot, with its old cistern and NPS sign on the banks of the river. Even if you are not staying overnight at Lopez River Campsite, it is a good spot to have lunch, stretch your legs, explore, write in your journal, or pleasantly idle away some time, waiting for a high-tide landing in Everglades City. On occasion, we have stopped here to brew a second cup of coffee and simply relax.

SECTION 4/R

MARKER 123/MARKER 107

Marker 123: N25° 48.050' W81° 17.363'
Marker 107: N25° 44.844' W81° 14.987'
Estimated paddling distance: 4.5 miles

NORTH TO SOUTH: Marker 123 to Marker 107

From marker 123 continue your paddle south down Sunday Bay. You will see marker 121 as the bay narrows toward its south end,

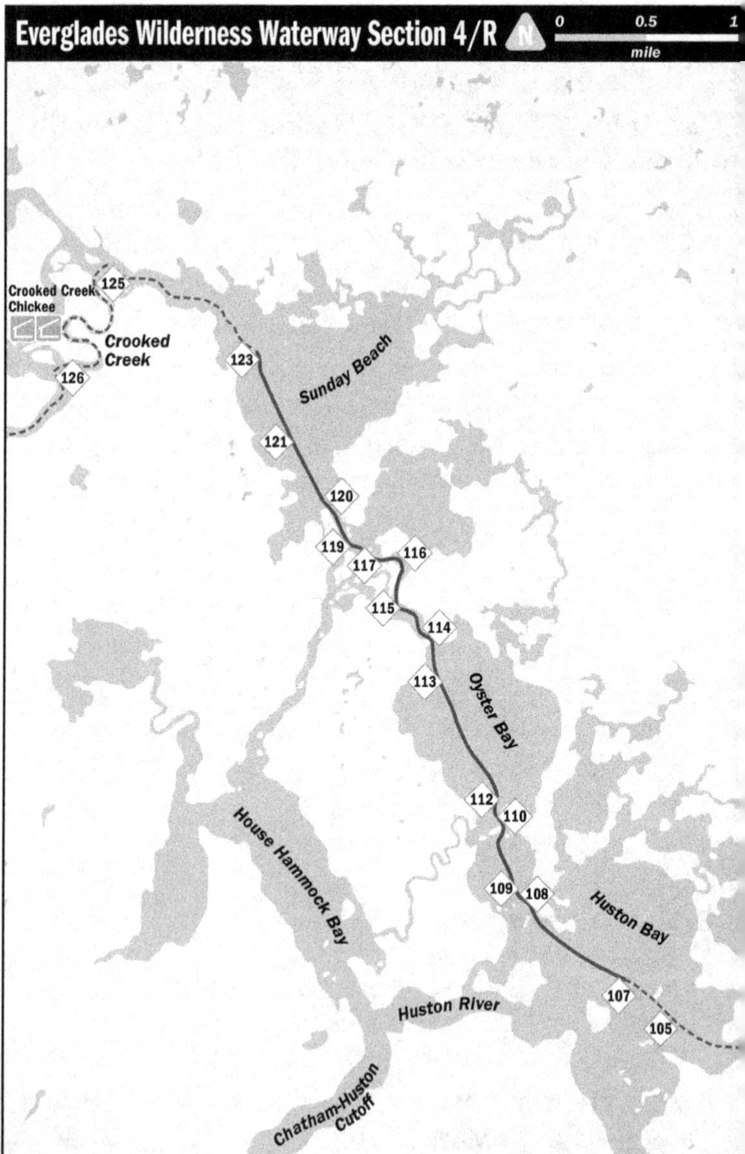
Everglades Wilderness Waterway Section 4/R
N
0
0.5
1
mile
Crooked Creek
Chickee
125
Crooked
Creek
126
123
Sunday Beach
121
120
119
117
116
115
114
113
Oyster Bay
112
110
109
108
Huston Bay
House Hammock Bay
107
105
Huston River
Chatham-Huston
Cutoff

and you will pass in quick succession markers 120, 119, 117, 116, 115, and 114, at which point you will enter Oyster Bay.

A word about mangroves: It's impossible to differentiate one mangrove island from another when you are out on the water. (It would be easier if you were looking down from an airplane.) Actually, many mangrove islands look just like part of the shoreline until you get close to them and realize they are islands. (Also see "Mangrove," on page 253.)

Pass marker 113 and head in a southeasterly direction across Oyster Bay, where you will see marker 112, followed by marker 110. Paddle south to marker 109 and then to 108 at the entrance to Huston Bay.

Continuing in a more easterly direction into Huston Bay, you will soon spot marker 107, located next to an island with a tidy red boathouse on stilts on the shore. This cabin, locally known as the Nauti Buoy, is the last private inholding in the park, and boaters are not allowed to land here.

SOUTH TO NORTH: Marker 107 to Marker 123

Paddle past marker 107, and you'll see the barn-board red boathouse on stilts—the last private property in the park. You are not permitted to land here, so make a northerly curve to markers 108 and 109. Paddle the lower portion of Oyster Bay, passing markers 110 and 112.

Continue in a northerly direction across Oyster Bay to marker 113 and then 114, which marks the channel to Sunday Bay. Paddle north, west, and north again, passing easy-to-spot markers 115, 116, 117, and 119.

At marker 120, you will enter the south end of Sunday Bay. Paddle in a northerly direction, passing marker 121 and then 123.

SECTION 5/Q

MARKER 107/THE WATSON PLACE OR SWEETWATER CHICKEE

Marker 107: N25° 44.844' W81° 14.987'
The Watson Place: N25° 42.551' W81° 14.737'
Sweetwater Chickee: N25° 44.617' W81° 12.685'
Estimated paddling distance, marker 107/The Watson Place: 4 miles
Estimated paddling distance, marker 107/Sweetwater Chickee: 4.5 miles

NORTH TO SOUTH: Marker 107 to The Watson Place or Sweetwater Chickee

Continue across Huston Bay to marker 105 and then to 103 at the entrance to Last Huston Bay. Last Huston Bay stretches out far to your left (east), so stay close to the west side of the bay, passing marker 102 that you will see out in the water.

As you leave Last Huston Bay, use caution. The Huston and Chatham rivers course from bays to the Gulf of Mexico, and if you hit the tides at the wrong time, the crosscurrents can be difficult to paddle, particularly in areas with narrow channels and shallow oyster beds. Often, we have paddled smoothly over this section, but once we had to step into the stream and pull our boat through the current until we reached a point at which we could paddle against it. Be sure to put on your water shoes if you must get into the water. This section of the Waterway has extensive oyster beds, and oyster shells are sharp—and can be dangerous, as noted in "Paddling Conditions," on page 6.

If you intend to camp at The Watson Place, turn right (west) at marker 100 onto the Chatham River. The Watson Place is approximately 1.5 miles downriver on your right. Do *not* follow the channel that branches off to the right about 1 mile down the Chatham, as it will lead you back to Huston Bay. Instead, continue on to The Watson Place, 0.5 mile farther down the main channel

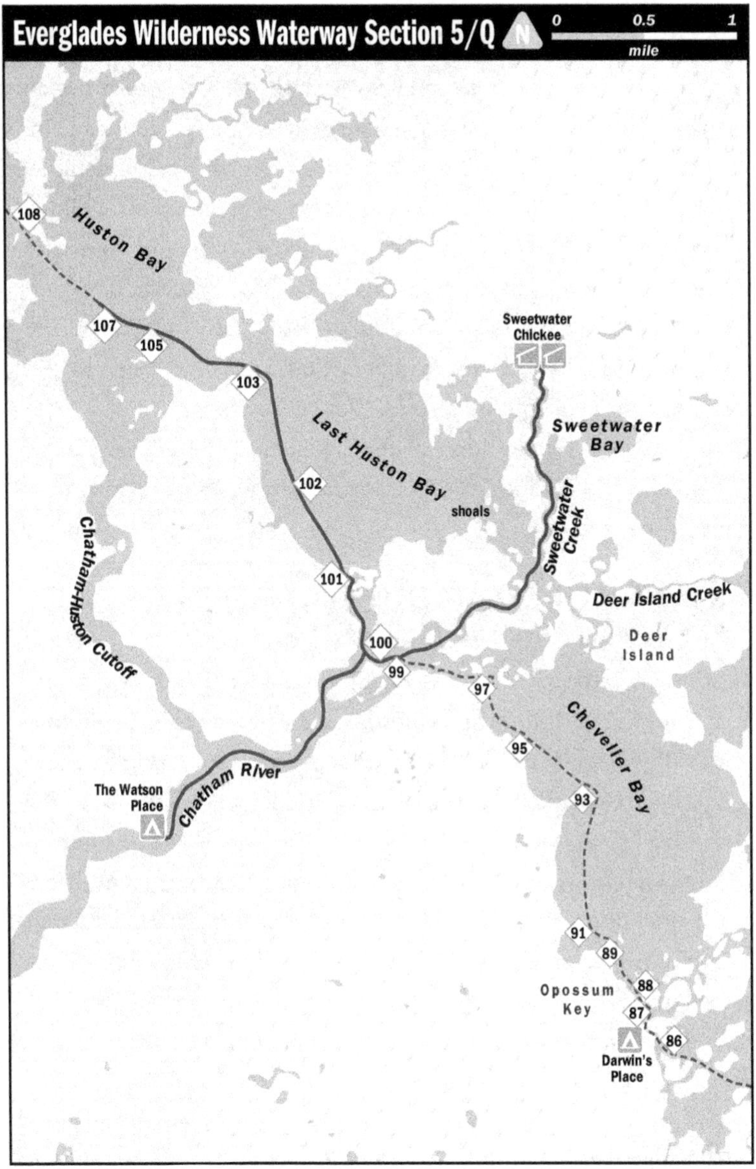
Everglades Wilderness Waterway Section 5/Q
N
0
0.5
1
mile
108
Huston Bay
107
105
103
Last Huston Bay
102
shoals
Sweetwater Chickee
Sweetwater Bay
Sweetwater Creek
101
100
99
97
Deer Island Creek
Deer Island
Chatham-Huston Cutoff
Chevelier Bay
95
93
The Watson Place
Chatham River
91
89
88
Opossum Key
87
86
Darwin's Place

of the Chatham on the right (west) bank. In the morning, backtrack northeast up the Chatham River to marker 100.

If you plan to camp at Sweetwater Chickee, turn left at marker 100, leave the marked Waterway, and head northeast. In about 1 mile you will come to a wide cross channel. Continue northeast across the channel to enter Sweetwater Creek. Follow Sweetwater Creek about a mile, staying consistently to your left, until you arrive at Sweetwater Chickee. Have patience, use your map and compass skills, and follow the map that accompanies this section. You'll know you're getting close when you begin to see a few cabbage palms.

Note: The location of the chickee can be a bit misleading on the NOAA chart. Look for the tiny line on the map that marks its spot.

SOUTH TO NORTH: Sweetwater Chickee or The Watson Place to Marker 107

From Sweetwater Chickee, paddle southwest to the Waterway and marker 100, turn right (north), and paddle into Last Huston Bay. If you stayed at The Watson Place, retrace your paddle up the Chatham to marker 100, turn left, and paddle north into Last Huston Bay. Use caution as you paddle the passage into Last Huston Bay. The Chatham and Huston rivers are strongly influenced by the tides from the Gulf of Mexico, and crosscurrents can be difficult to paddle, particularly where channels narrow. If you need to step into the water to pull your boat through the current, be sure to wear shoes to protect your feet from sharp oyster shells.

(An alternative route from The Watson Place into Huston Bay is to retrace your paddle northeast and take the Chatham-Huston Cutoff on your left. It is the channel that branched off the Chatham just before you arrived at The Watson Place. This route

Syrup kettle at The Watson Place

will take you to the south end of Huston Bay, where you will continue your journey northward, watching for marker 105.)

Continue on to markers (sitting out in the water) 102 and 103. At marker 103, round the bend to your left, heading northwest into Huston Bay toward marker 105 and then marker 107.

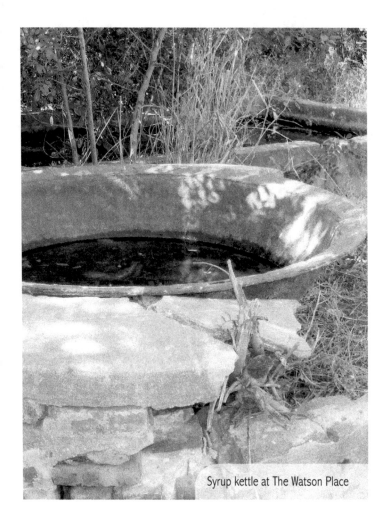

SECTION 6/P

THE WATSON PLACE OR SWEETWATER CHICKEE/MARKER 79

The Watson Place: N25° 42.551' W81° 14.737'
Sweetwater Chickee: N25° 44.617' W81° 12.685'
Marker 79: N25° 41.000' W81° 11.459'
Estimated paddling distance, The Watson Place/marker 79: 5 miles
Estimated paddling distance, Sweetwater Chickee/marker 79: 5 miles

NORTH TO SOUTH: The Watson Place or Sweetwater Chickee to Marker 79

If you stayed at The Watson Place, backtrack northeastward up the Chatham River to marker 100 and turn east (right).

If you stayed at Sweetwater Chickee, paddle back along the passage you took when you came to the chickee to marker 100. Turn left and paddle easterly until you reach marker 97.

At marker 97 you will enter Chevelier Bay (see page 247). Stay to the right (west) side of the bay, passing markers 95, 93, and 91. Close to the shore, you will pass some islands on your left (east) and come to marker 88, which marks the entrance to the channel that leads to marker 87 and passes Darwin's Place, a ground campsite, on Opossum Key on your right. You will see the tabby remains of Darwin's home (see "Tabby," on page 262).

Continue southeast, crossing the western side of Cannon Bay and passing markers 86 and 85. At marker 83 you will turn right (south) and enter narrow Tarpon Bay and pass markers 81 and 79.

SOUTH TO NORTH: Marker 79 to Sweetwater Chickee or The Watson Place

Paddle north to pass markers 79 and 81, where the bay funnels north up a channel to marker 83 at the entrance to Cannon Bay. Paddle by a small island, keeping marker 85 on your left, and cross the southwestern part of Cannon Bay, leaving the bulk of the bay

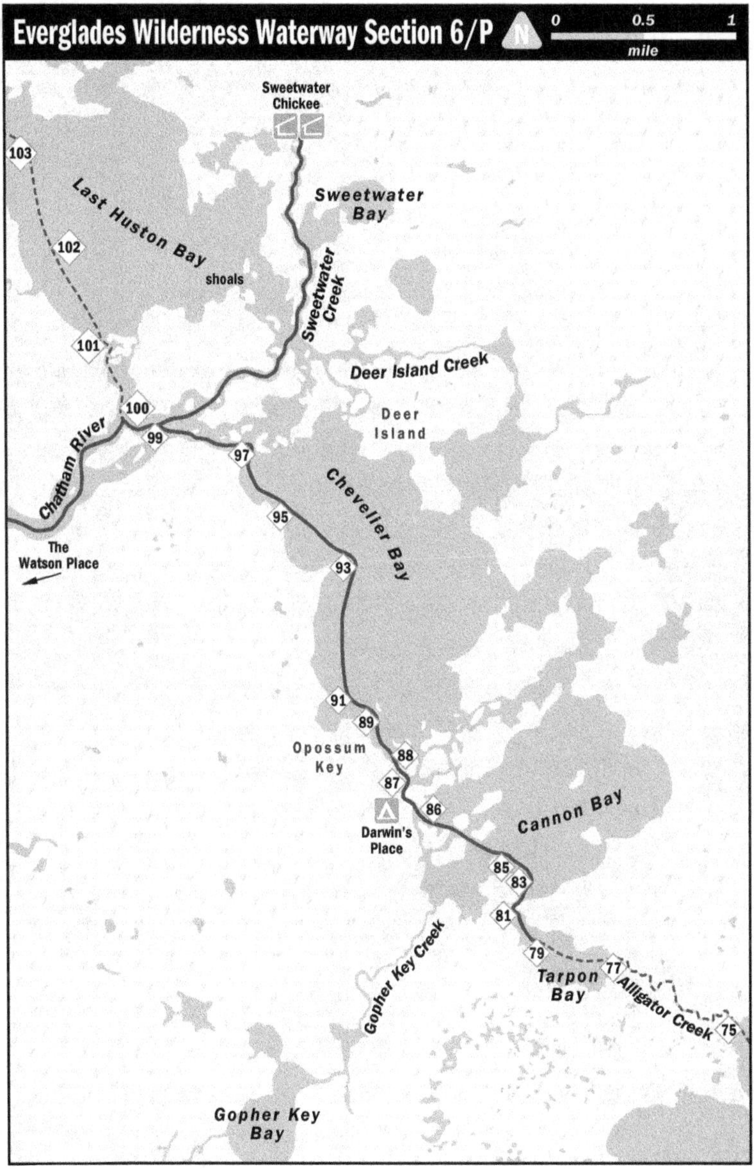
Everglades Wilderness Waterway Section 6/P
N
0
0.5
1
mile
Sweetwater Chickee
103
Last Huston Bay
Sweetwater Bay
102
shoals
Sweetwater Creek
101
Deer Island Creek
100
Deer Island
Chatham River
99
97
Chevelier Bay
95
The Watson Place
93
91
89
Opossum Key
88
87
86
Darwin's Place
Cannon Bay
85
83
81
Gopher Key Creek
79
77
Tarpon Bay
Alligator Creek
75
Gopher Key Bay

to your right. Travel between two pairs of islands to marker 86, and enter the channel that passes Darwin's Place on Opossum Key to your left. Darwin's Place is a ground site, easy to spot because of the NPS sign, the privy, and the homestead's tabby foundations (see "Darwin's Place," on page 219, and "Tabby," on page 262).

A short distance farther, pass markers 87, 88, and 89 as you head north into Chevelier Bay. Look for marker 91 on your left (west) and head north along the western shoreline of the bay. Again, the largest part of the bay is to your right. Marker 93 stands on a peninsula reaching out into the bay; when you pass this point, turn in a more westerly direction toward markers 95 and 97. As in all of the larger bays, conditions can be rough here if the wind is up. If this is the case, you might find some protection by staying near the shoreline. You may have to tack, paddling into the waves so that they don't catch you broadside. At marker 97 head west and follow the left shoreline.

If you are heading for Sweetwater Chickee, turn right at marker 99, where the Chatham River comes in on the left (west). Follow the channel about 1 mile northeast until you come to a large cross-channel. Paddle to the other side where Sweetwater Creek opens directly to the northeast. Some paddlers report having difficulty locating Sweetwater Chickee. But if you just follow the creek about a mile, keeping left, you will arrive at the chickee.

If you are heading for The Watson Place, paddle north and turn left (west) at marker 100; paddle 1.5 miles down the Chatham River. A mile down, you will pass a channel branching off to your right, but stay on the main channel; after another 0.5 mile you will spot The Watson Place to your right.

SECTION 7/0

MARKER 79/PLATE CREEK CHICKEE OR LOSTMANS FIVE CAMPSITE

Marker 79: N25° 41.000' W81° 11.459'
Plate Creek Chickee: N25° 38.459' W81° 08.949'
Lostmans Five Campsite: N25° 38.039' W81° 08.551'
Estimated paddling distance, marker 79/Plate Creek: 6 miles
Estimated paddling distance, marker 79/Lostmans Five Campsite: 7 miles

NORTH TO SOUTH: Marker 79 to Plate Creek Chickee or Lostmans Five Campsite

From marker 79 cross Tarpon Bay to the entrance to Alligator Creek. The last few times we paddled the Waterway, marker 77 was missing from the entrance to Alligator Creek. The creek is not difficult to find, however, as Tarpon Bay funnels into it. Alligator Creek is lovely, narrow, and winding. Pioneer Totch Brown, in his memoir, *Totch: A Life in the Everglades,* wrote of his dad's claim that Gator Bay Creek got its name from an alligator nobody could kill. Before laws that prohibited alligator hunting were passed in the 1960s, many residents of the Everglades made their living by capturing these reptiles, skinning them, and profiting from the sale of the hides. Alligators (see page 245) were brought to the brink of extinction before these laws were passed, but the population has rebounded dramatically. You will likely see alligators here or elsewhere on your Waterway trip.

Alligator Creek opens into Alligator Bay at marker 75. Paddle in a southeasterly direction and pass marker 73 out in the water. Continue on a more easterly course, leaving the expanse of Alligator Bay to your right (southwest).

Look for marker 72, a bit difficult to see tucked near the mangrove shoreline, and then enter Dad's Bay. Stay near the left (east) side of the bay, passing markers 70 and 68 and a

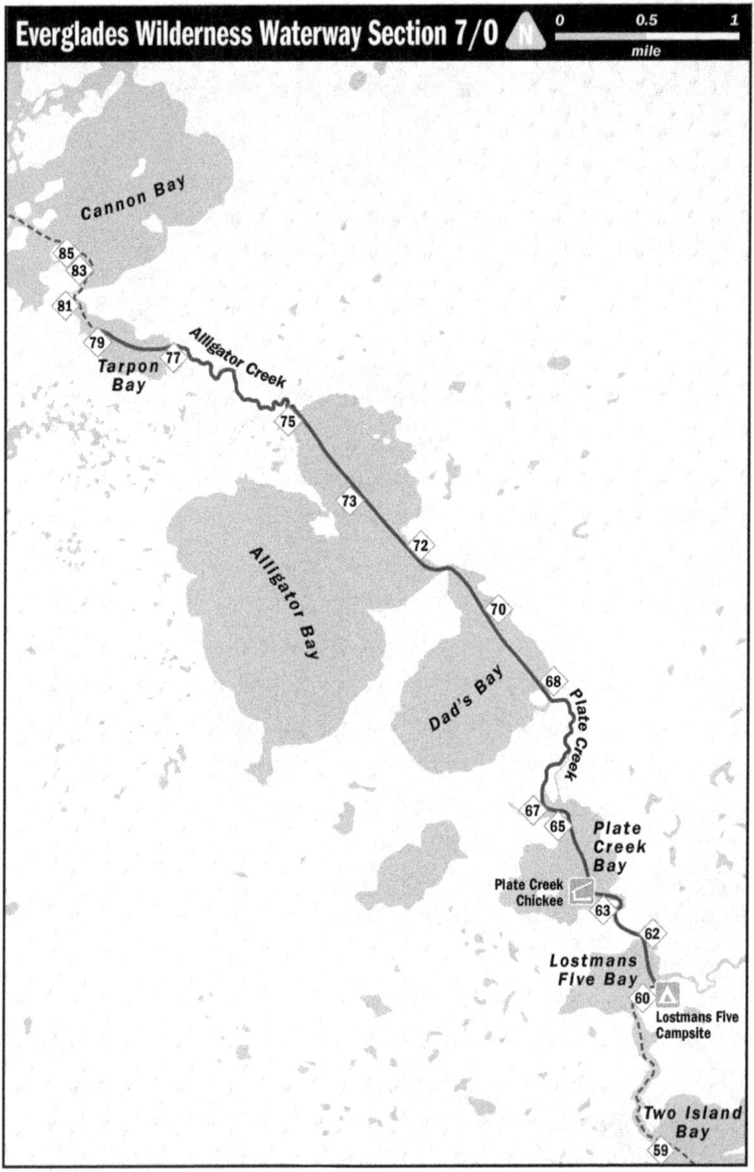
Everglades Wilderness Waterway Section 7/0
N
0
0.5
1
mile
Cannon Bay
85
83
81
79
Tarpon Bay
77
Alligator Creek
75
73
72
Alligator Bay
70
Dad's Bay
68
Plate Creek
67
65
Plate Creek Bay
Plate Creek Chickee
63
62
Lostmans Five Bay
60
Lostmans Five Campsite
Two Island Bay
59

NO WAKE sign that mark the entrance to Plate Creek. Plate Creek (see page 234) is narrow and lined with mangroves, palms, and air plants. The water is a clear amber color, and you can watch the fish swim by.

Markers 67 and 65 signal the entrance to Plate Creek Bay. Cross Plate Creek Bay in a southeasterly direction and you will spot Plate Creek Chickee to your right, at the end of an island west of marker 63.

If you are heading for Lostmans Five Campsite, paddle the channel between markers 63 and 62 and then south across Lostmans Five Bay to Lostmans Five Campsite near marker 60.

SOUTH TO NORTH: Lostmans Five Campsite or Plate Creek Chickee to Marker 79

If you stayed at Lostmans Five Campsite, travel north across the bay to marker 62 and enter the channel that leads into Plate Creek Bay and marker 63. Plate Creek Chickee lies west of marker 63, so if you stayed there, travel east to marker 63.

From either point of origin, paddle north across Plate Creek Bay, from marker 63 to 65, the main body of Plate Creek Bay to your left (west). With sharp eyes or binoculars, you can spot marker 65 from the Plate Creek Chickee. The marker stands at the entrance to Plate Creek, which is narrow, lined with mangroves, the occasional palm tree, and air plants. It flows clear and amber-colored, and you can look for fish swimming below your boat.

Follow this channel to Dad's Bay, a NO WAKE sign, and marker 68. Again the body of the bay is to your left (west), so paddle along the eastern shore to marker 70. Dad's Bay narrows soon after, and you will pass into Alligator Bay.

At the point where marker 72 appears on your right, head in a northwesterly direction across the northern part of Alligator Bay, paddling past marker 73 in the middle of the bay, and then marker

75 at the beginning of Alligator Creek. The creek is two boats wide; is winding; is lined with mangroves, buttonwoods, and air plants; and offers a good chance of seeing an alligator. The pioneer Totch Brown, in his memoir, *Totch: A Life in the Everglades,* suggested that the creek was named for an alligator nobody could kill. Travel the creek until you come out onto small and lovely Tarpon Bay. (The last times we've paddled, marker 77 has been missing from the exit from Alligator Creek. By the time you get there, it may have been replaced.) Paddle the length of the bay, passing marker 79.

SECTION 8/N

PLATE CREEK CHICKEE OR LOSTMANS FIVE CAMPSITE/MARKER 49

Plate Creek Chickee: N25° 38.459' W81° 08.949'
Lostmans Five Campsite: N25° 38.039' W81° 08.551'
Marker 49: N25° 34.561' W81° 07.438'
Estimated paddling distance, Plate Creek Chickee/marker 49: 6.5 miles
Estimated paddling distance, Lostmans Five Campsite/marker 49: 5.5 miles

NORTH TO SOUTH: Plate Creek Chickee or Lostmans Five Campsite to Marker 49

Leave Plate Creek Chickee, paddle the channel between markers 63 and 62, and head south across Lostmans Five Bay to Lostmans Five Campsite, near marker 60. If leaving from Lostmans Five Campsite, you are already at your starting point.

At marker 60, enter the passage leading from Lostmans Five Bay south to Two Island Bay, where you pass marker 59. Head southeast across the bay to marker 58. Marker 58 can be a little tricky to find traveling north to south. Follow the right shoreline and you will come to the marker. On a sunny day you can also look for the change in coloration of the trees to help yourself see the passage. A contrast of dark and light will suggest a gap in the shoreline, which marks the channel to Onion Key Bay.

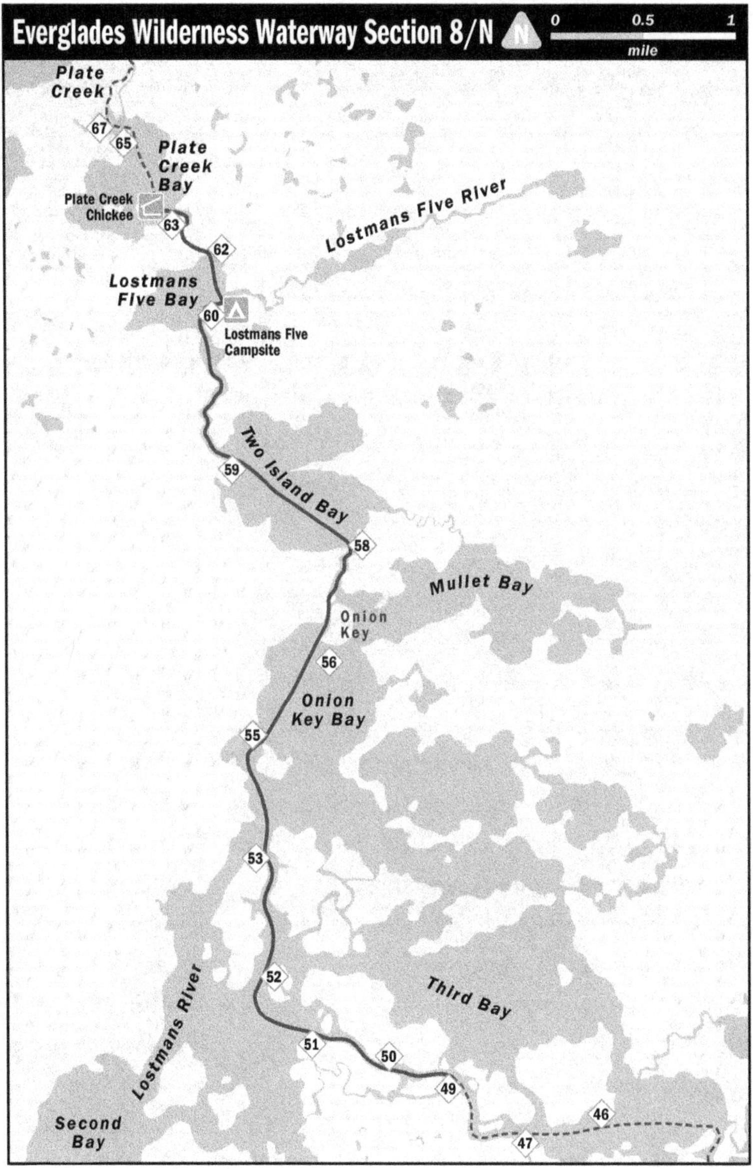
Everglades Wilderness Waterway Section 8/N
N
0
0.5
1
mile
Plate Creek
67
65
Plate Creek Bay
Plate Creek Chickee
63
62
Lostmans Five River
Lostmans Five Bay
60
Lostmans Five Campsite
59
Two Island Bay
58
Mullet Bay
Onion Key
56
Onion Key Bay
55
53
52
Third Bay
Lostmans River
51
50
49
46
47
Second Bay

Pass Onion Key (see page 257), which is a shell mound to your left (east). This spot used to be a campsite but is now closed to the public. Pass marker 56 on your left and cross Onion Key Bay, following the western shore. Paddle southwest past the island in the bay and then southeast to marker 53. Head south between mangrove islands and then southeast toward marker 51 and into a channel between large mangrove islands. Paddle in an easterly direction down the channel to marker 49.

SOUTH TO NORTH: Marker 49 to Lostmans Five Campsite or Plate Creek Chickee

Paddle northwest up the channel from marker 49, passing marker 50 and then 51 at the end of the channel. Continue traveling northwest to marker 52 and then north to 53. (Use your charts to help you through this area if markers are missing.)

You are now entering Onion Key Bay. Stay to the western shoreline of the bay, continuing northeast to marker 56 next to Onion Key, a little shell mound on your right. Pass the mound and enter the channel to reach Two Island Bay and marker 58.

Once in Two Island Bay, turn left and head across the bay in a northwesterly direction. You will pass a peninsula jutting out to your right and a smaller one to your left. You will pass marker 59 to your left as you approach the exit from Two Island Bay.

Pass marker 59 and enter the channel that leads to Lostmans Five Bay. If you are paddling to the Lostmans Five Campsite, look for marker 60 to the north; the campsite sits on the shore, just beyond the marker. In the morning, travel north across the bay to marker 62.

If you are paddling to the Plate Creek Chickee, head north across Lostmans Five Bay to marker 62, which indicates the channel to Plate Creek Bay. The chickee is visible inside the bay, west of marker 63.

SECTION 9/M

MARKER 49/EAST END OF BIG LOSTMANS BAY

Marker 49: N25° 34.561' W81° 07.438'
East End of Big Lostmans Bay (marker 38): N25° 34.013' W81° 04.174'
Estimated paddling distance: 3.5 miles

NORTH TO SOUTH:
Marker 49 to East End of Big Lostmans Bay

On this leg of your journey, you will be traveling more west to east than north to south. From marker 49, follow the channel as it turns south, then east into an unnamed bay, and pass markers 47 and 46. Be alert for marker 45, which is a little hard to spot on the mangrove shoreline. If the wind is out of the east, this can be a strenuous paddle.

At marker 45, the Waterway takes a sharp turn south to marker 44, which signals the entrance to Big Lostmans Bay. Continue southeast to marker 42 and keep east following the southern shore of Big Lostmans Bay, passing a couple of entrances to Rodgers River Bay on your right. You will pass markers 41 and 39 on your right. Cross the entrance to Rodgers River Bay at marker 39. Paddle northeast to the east end of Big Lostmans Bay (marker 38 on the charts). At this point you will either continue east into Lostmans Creek to go to Willy Willy Campsite, or turn right (southeast) and follow a channel across the easterly end of Rodgers River Bay to go to Rodgers River Chickee.

SOUTH TO NORTH:
East End of Big Lostmans Bay to Marker 49

At the east end of Big Lostmans Bay (marker 38), head due west across the southern portion of the bay. You will pass marker 39 and then marker 41 on your left. Continue west until you pass

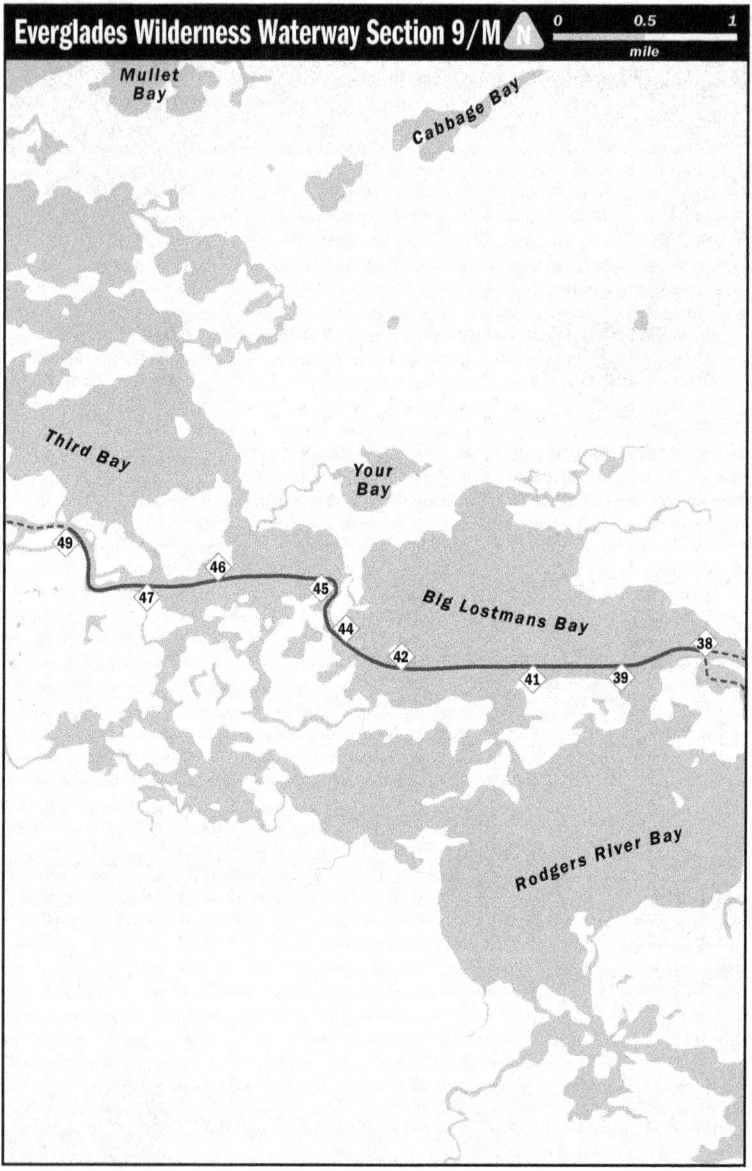
Everglades Wilderness Waterway Section 9/M
N
0
0.5
1
mile
Mullet Bay
Cabbage Bay
Third Bay
Your Bay
Big Lostmans Bay
Rodgers River Bay
49
46
47
45
44
42
41
39
38

marker 42, and then turn in a more northerly direction to marker 44. Paddle the channel to marker 45 and west across an unnamed bay to marker 47. Enter the channel and paddle west, then north, and then west again to marker 49, where you can see an opening to Third Bay on your right.

SECTION 10/L

EAST END OF BIG LOSTMANS BAY (MARKER 38)/WILLY WILLY CAMPSITE OR RODGERS RIVER CHICKEE

East End of Big Lostmans Bay: N25° 34.013' W81° 04.174'
Willy Willy Campsite: N25° 34.840' W81° 03.333'
Rodgers River Chickee: N25° 32.138' W81° 03.742'
Estimated paddling distance, East End of Big Lostmans Bay/Willy Willy Campsite: 2.5 miles
Estimated paddling distance, East End of Big Lostmans Bay/Rodgers River Chickee: 3.5 miles

NORTH TO SOUTH:
East End of Big Lostmans Bay to Willy Willy Campsite or Rodgers River Chickee

If you intend to camp at Willy Willy Campsite, continue east from the end of Big Lostmans Bay (marker 38) into Lostmans Creek.

Follow the left shore of Lostmans Creek and take the third channel left into Rocky Creek, paddle about 1 mile, and then take another left into Rocky Creek Bay. The Willy Willy Campsite will be to the right soon after you enter the bay. Retrace this route in the morning.

If you plan to camp at Rodgers River Chickee, turn right (southeast) at the east end of Big Lostmans Bay (marker 38) and head into the channel that skirts the eastern edge of Rodgers River Bay. Use your charts to navigate this tricky section. Look for marker 37 in the channel. *This marker is not indicated on the NOAA or Waterproof navigational charts.* You will cross the

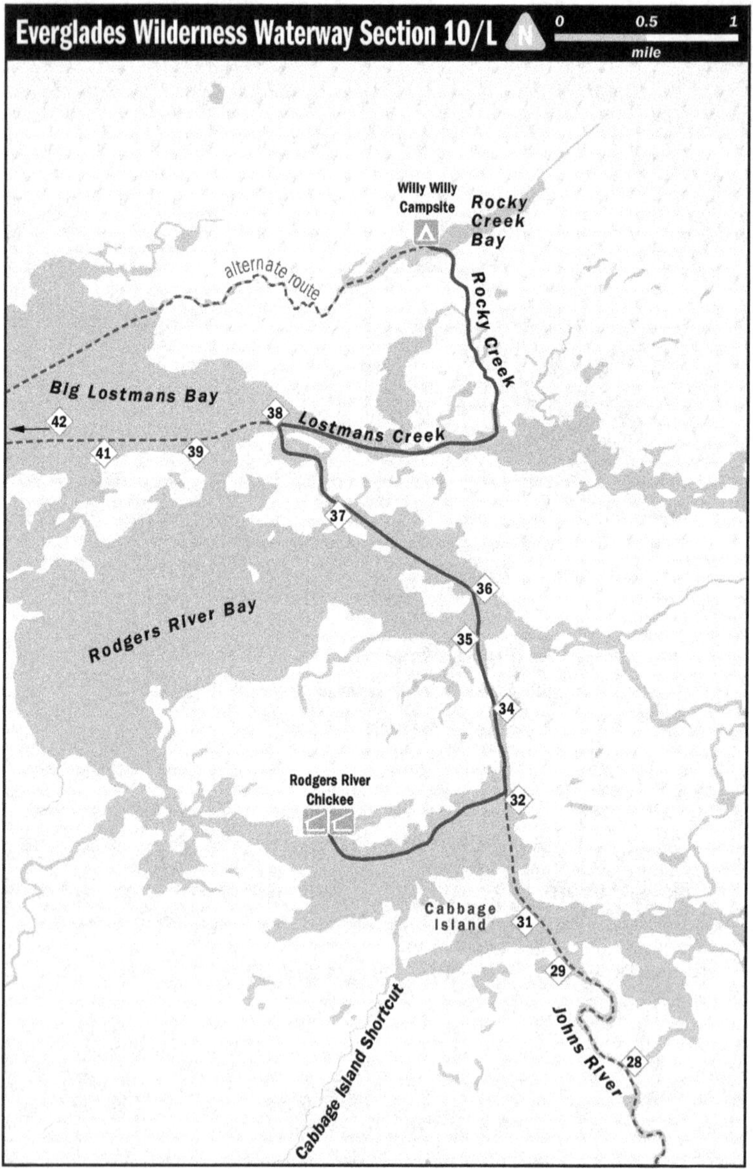
Everglades Wilderness Waterway Section 10/L
N
0
0.5
1
mile
Willy Willy Campsite
Rocky Creek Bay
Rocky Creek
alternate route
Big Lostmans Bay
Lostmans Creek
42
41
39
38
37
36
35
34
32
31
29
28
Rodgers River Bay
Rodgers River Chickee
Cabbage Island
Cabbage Island Shortcut
Johns River

northeast end of Rodgers River Bay. Paddle southeast and then south when you see marker 35. Pass markers 35, 34, and 32.

At marker 32, turn right (west) into the southeastern portion of Rodgers River Bay (see page 258).

The Rodgers River Chickee will be past seven spits of land, on the right (northern) shore of this part of the bay, about a mile from marker 32. *Note:* Current navigational charts do not mark the location of this chickee accurately, as it is farther from marker 32 than indicated.

SOUTH TO NORTH:
Rodgers River Chickee or Willy Willy Campsite to East End of Big Lostmans Bay

Leaving Rodgers River Chickee in the morning, head east into the sun, and paddle back to marker 32. Turn left (north) and pass markers 34 and 35. This is a tricky spot to navigate, and markers may be missing, so use your charts. At marker 35 you will skirt the eastern edge of Rodgers River Bay. Stay to the right (eastern) side of the channel and travel generally northwest, jogging west, north, west, and north. You will spot Big Lostmans Bay to your left (west) as you come out of this channel.

If you stayed at Willy Willy Campsite, retrace your route in the morning to Big Lostmans Bay, or continue west down Rocky Creek Bay and into the narrow channel that leads to Big Lostmans Bay. This shortcut will save you time and allows you to paddle past a short stretch on your right (north) that is lined with sawgrass. Because mangroves predominate along the Waterway, this is a real treat. When you enter Big Lostmans Bay, marker 41 will be south of your position, so be sure to look for marker 42 to the southwest and proceed northward from there.

SECTION 11/K

WILLY WILLY CAMPSITE OR RODGERS RIVER CHICKEE/MARKER 26

Willy Willy Campsite: N25° 34.840' W81° 03.333'
Rodgers River Chickee: N25° 32.138' W81° 03.742'
WW marker 26: N25° 30.097' W81° 02.434'
Estimated paddling distance, Willy Willy Campsite/ marker 26: 7.5 miles
Estimated paddling distance, Rodgers River Chickee/ marker 26: 4.5 miles

NORTH TO SOUTH: Willy Willy Campsite or Rodgers River Chickee to Marker 26

If you stayed at Willy Willy Campsite, return to the east end of Big Lostmans Bay and turn left (southeast), heading into the channel that skirts the eastern edge of Rodgers River Bay. Travel on the *eastern* side of the islands in the bay. When you pass the large last island, head south into the channel and pass markers 35, 34, and 32. This is a tricky spot to navigate, and some of the markers may be missing, so use your charts.

Note: We provide the GPS coordinates for both markers 36 and 37 in Appendix 7, on page 288.

If you stayed at Rodgers River Chickee, travel east to return to marker 32. From marker 32 paddle south to marker 31. Cabbage Island (see page 247) will be on your right (west). Continue south past marker 29, along the passage (called Johns River on the Waterproof Charts, unnamed on the NOAA charts) to Broad River Bay, which is really a wide place in the Broad River, at marker 26.

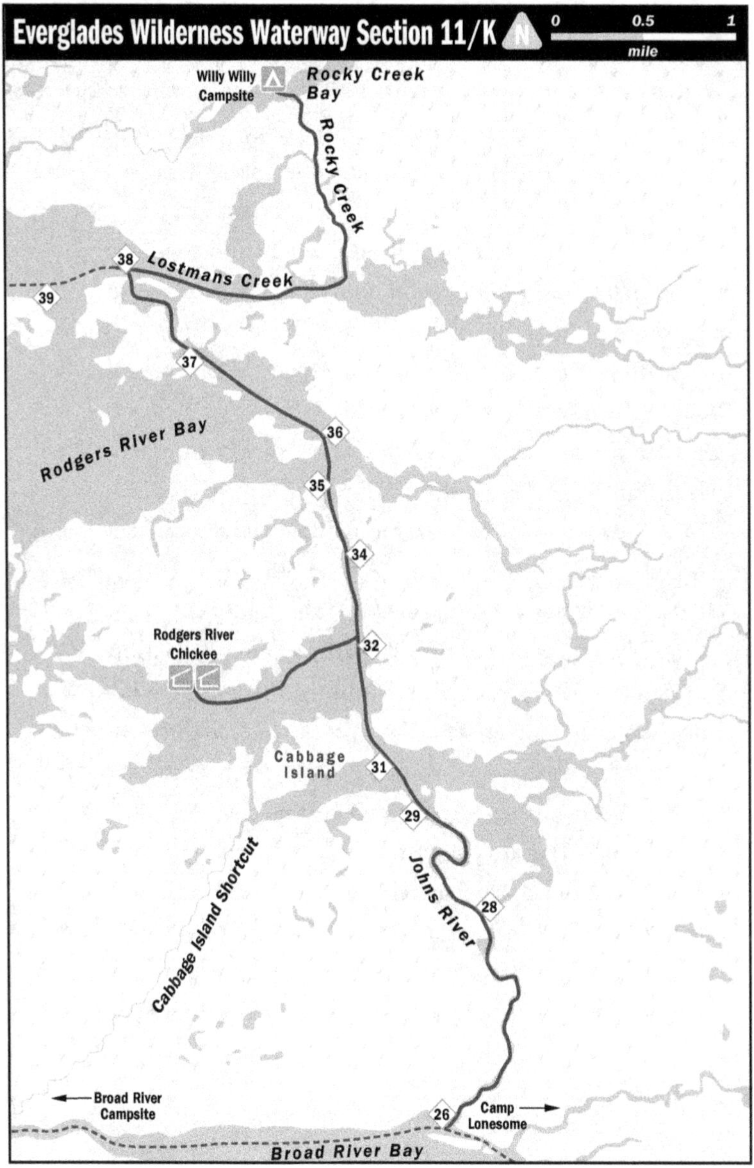
Everglades Wilderness Waterway Section 11/K
N
0
0.5
1
mile
Willy Willy Campsite
Rocky Creek Bay
Rocky Creek
38
39
Lostmans Creek
37
36
Rodgers River Bay
35
34
Rodgers River Chickee
32
Cabbage Island
31
29
Johns River
28
Cabbage Island Shortcut
Broad River Campsite
26
Camp Lonesome
Broad River Bay

SOUTH TO NORTH: Marker 26 to Rodgers River Chickee or Willy Willy Campsite

At marker 26, turn north leaving Broad River Bay through Johns River (not named on the NOAA charts). Stay to the left when the river branches. You will cross an unnamed bay at marker 29. Pass marker 31, and enter the channel with Cabbage Island to your left (west). As you pass Cabbage Island, continue north, staying close to the right (eastern) shoreline until you reach marker 32. (See page 247 for more on Cabbage Island.)

If you plan to stay at Rodgers River Chickee, turn left (west) at marker 32 and head into the bay. The Rodgers River Chickee will be about 1 mile down on the right (northern) shore of this part of the bay, past 7 small projections of land.

Note: The location of the Rodgers River Chickee is not marked accurately on the NOAA or Waterproof navigational charts; it is farther west into the bay than indicated.

If you plan to stay at Willy Willy Campsite, continue north past markers 32, 34, and 35. Continue north and then northwest along the channel that skirts the east side of Rodgers River Bay. Check your charts, as this section is tricky to navigate and markers have been missing. At the end of this channel you will see Big Lostmans Bay to your left. Turn right and enter Lostmans Creek. Take the third channel on your left (north), and paddle into Rocky Creek for about 1 mile until it opens onto Rocky Creek Bay. Turn left down Rocky Creek Bay and you will, after a short paddle, spot Willy Willy Campsite on your right.

SECTION 12/J

MARKER 26/CAMP LONESOME OR BROAD RIVER CAMPSITE

Marker 26: N25° 30.097' W81° 02.434'
Camp Lonesome: N25° 29.292' W80° 59.994'
Broad River Campsite: N25° 28.748' W81° 08.534'
Estimated paddling distance, marker 26/Camp Lonesome: 3.5 miles
Estimated paddling distance, marker 26/Broad River Campsite: 6.5 miles

NORTH TO SOUTH: Marker 26 to Camp Lonesome or Broad River Campsite

If you plan to stay at Camp Lonesome, a ground site, turn left (east) at marker 26 and follow the Broad River east to the campsite. Stay to the right (south) side of the Broad River because a number of small channels enter into the river from the left (north). Just after you pass the Wood River on your right, the Broad River will branch. Turn into the left (northeast) branch and you will soon see Camp Lonesome on the left bank of the river. You won't be able to see it until you're practically in front of it. In the morning, retrace your route to marker 26 and paddle west, then southwest, to the Broad River Campsite.

If you are bypassing Camp Lonesome to stay at the Broad River Campsite, turn right (west) at marker 26 into Broad River Bay, which funnels into the Broad River.

As you paddle southwest down the Broad River, you will not pass any markers for approximately 5 miles until you reach marker 25. Just before the marker, however, you will see the Broad River Campsite on the southern (left) shore of the Broad River. This ground site is a good place from which to start paddling The Nightmare in the morning, if the tides allow.

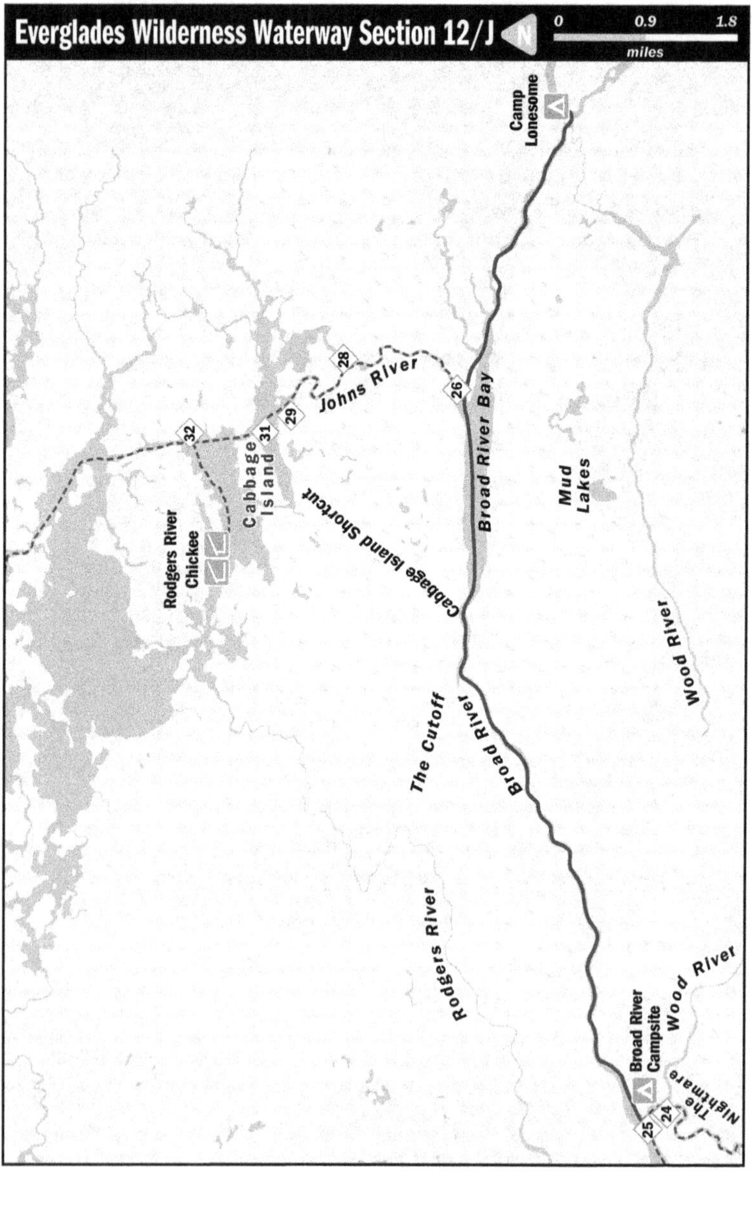
Everglades Wilderness Waterway Section 12/J
N
0
0.9
1.8
miles
Camp Lonesome
Johns River
28
26
29
31
32
Cabbage Island
Broad River Bay
Mud Lakes
Rodgers River Chickee
Cabbage Island Shortcut
Wood River
The Cutoff
Broad River
Rodgers River
Broad River Campsite
Wood River
The Nightmare
24
25

SOUTH TO NORTH: Broad River Campsite to Marker 26 or Camp Lonesome

From the Broad River Campsite, paddle northeast up the Broad River for approximately 4.5 miles, where the Broad River makes a sharp bend right (east) and in 0.5 mile widens into Broad River Bay. Travel about 1.5 miles along the bay, angling in a northeasterly direction to find marker 26 where you leave the bay. This channel is called Johns River on the Waterproof Charts; it is not named on the NOAA charts.

To Camp Lonesome, continue southeast for about 3 miles on the Broad beyond marker 26. Keep right, on the south side of the Broad River, to avoid being confused by small channels entering from the left (north). Immediately after the Wood River enters on the right, follow the left (northeast) branch of the Broad. Camp Lonesome will quickly appear on your left.

In the morning, follow the Broad River back the way you came and, once in Broad River Bay, look for marker 26 at the end of the island where the Broad River enters the bay. Turn right (north) into Johns River.

SECTION 13/I

BROAD RIVER CAMPSITE & HIGHLAND BEACH EXCURSION

Broad River Campsite: N25° 28.748' W81° 08.534'
Highland Beach: N25° 28.677' W81° 11.079'
Estimated paddling distance (round-trip): 8 miles

NORTH TO SOUTH and SOUTH TO NORTH: Broad River Campsite to Highland Beach to Broad River Campsite

The enticing option here is to spend time at Highland Beach. You may paddle over to it as an excursion from the Broad River

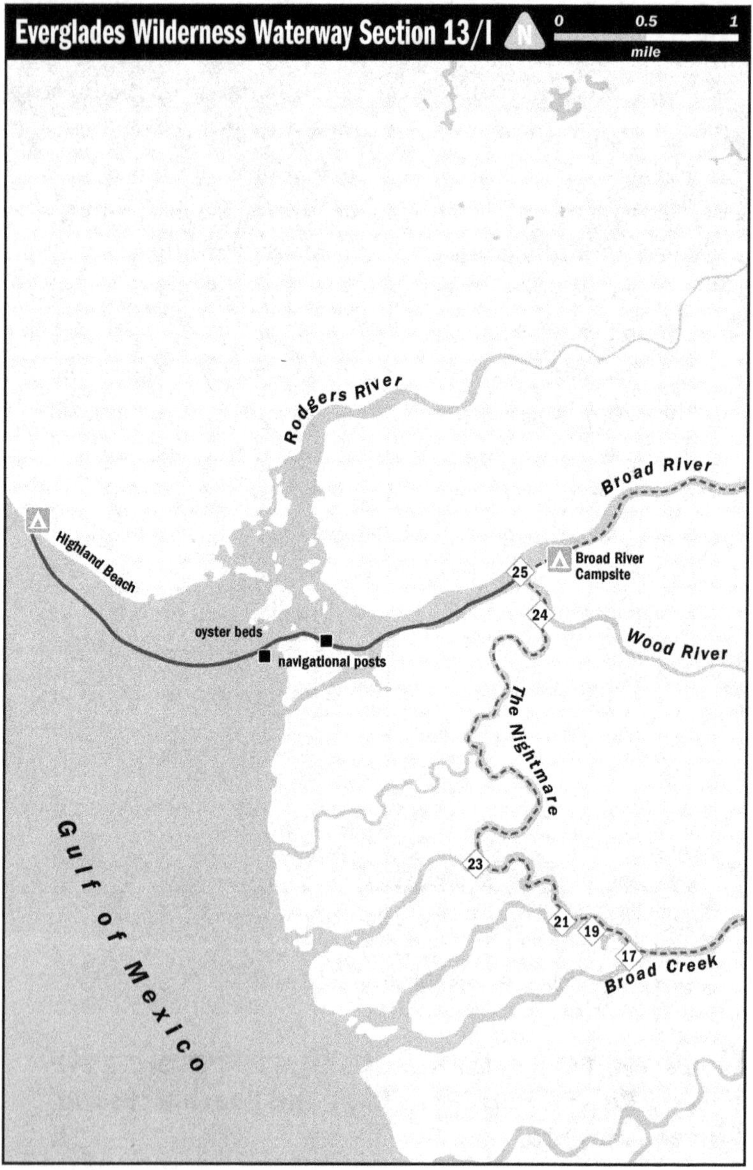
Everglades Wilderness Waterway Section 13/I
N
0
0.5
1
mile
Rodgers River
Broad River
Broad River Campsite
Highland Beach
25
24
Wood River
oyster beds
navigational posts
The Nightmare
Gulf of Mexico
23
21
19
17
Broad Creek

Campsite (or from nearby marker 25). Or you may want to spend a night on this Gulf of Mexico shore before or after doing The Nightmare. Either way, paddle westward on the Broad River until you reach the Gulf, watching for navigation markers at the left (south) side of the mouth of the river. These markers alert you to the channel that leads through the islands at the mouth of the river, a passage that helps you avoid the oyster beds. Once in the Gulf and clear of the oysters, turn right (north) and paddle up the coast.

Continue until you find any spot on the beach that suits you for stretching your legs, some beachcombing, or simply lazing about. You might even consider spending an extra day and night at Highland Beach. You will have a choice spot for watching the sun set into the tranquil horizon in this part of the world.

In the morning, retrace your paddle south along the Gulf and then east into the Broad River, carefully following the channel markers.

Highland Beach

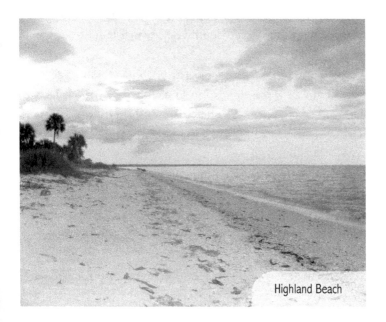

SECTION 14/H

BROAD RIVER CAMPSITE/HARNEY RIVER CHICKEE VIA THE NIGHTMARE

Broad River Campsite: N25° 28.748' W81° 08.534'
Harney River Chickee (marker 12): N25° 25.953' W81° 05.464'
Estimated paddling distance: 8.5 miles

NORTH TO SOUTH: Broad River Campsite to Harney River Chickee via The Nightmare

From the Broad River Campsite, paddle southwest on the Broad River a short distance to marker 25 on the left (south), indicating the entrance to the Wood River, which you will follow for a little more than 0.25 mile to its divergence at the entrance to The Nightmare.

Or, from Highland Beach, retrace your paddle south down the Gulf, and enter the Broad, heading eastward, where you will travel for about 1.5 miles to marker 25 on the right (south). Turn into the Wood River and you will shortly see marker 24 on your right (southwest), which indicates the start of The Nightmare.

Note: You cannot paddle The Nightmare at low tide. You will get stuck. If the tide is too low, either wait until the tide comes in or go out to the Gulf and paddle south to the Harney River, where you will turn left (east), continuing up the river to marker 12 and the Harney River Chickee.

With its narrow, twisting channel that is impossible to get through at low tide; confusing to navigate at extreme high tide; and crisscrossed by low mangrove branches, fallen trees, and spiderwebs at all tides and times, The Nightmare has certainly earned its name.

In spite of its challenges (and because of them), The Nightmare is lovely, with water the creamy color of café au lait and

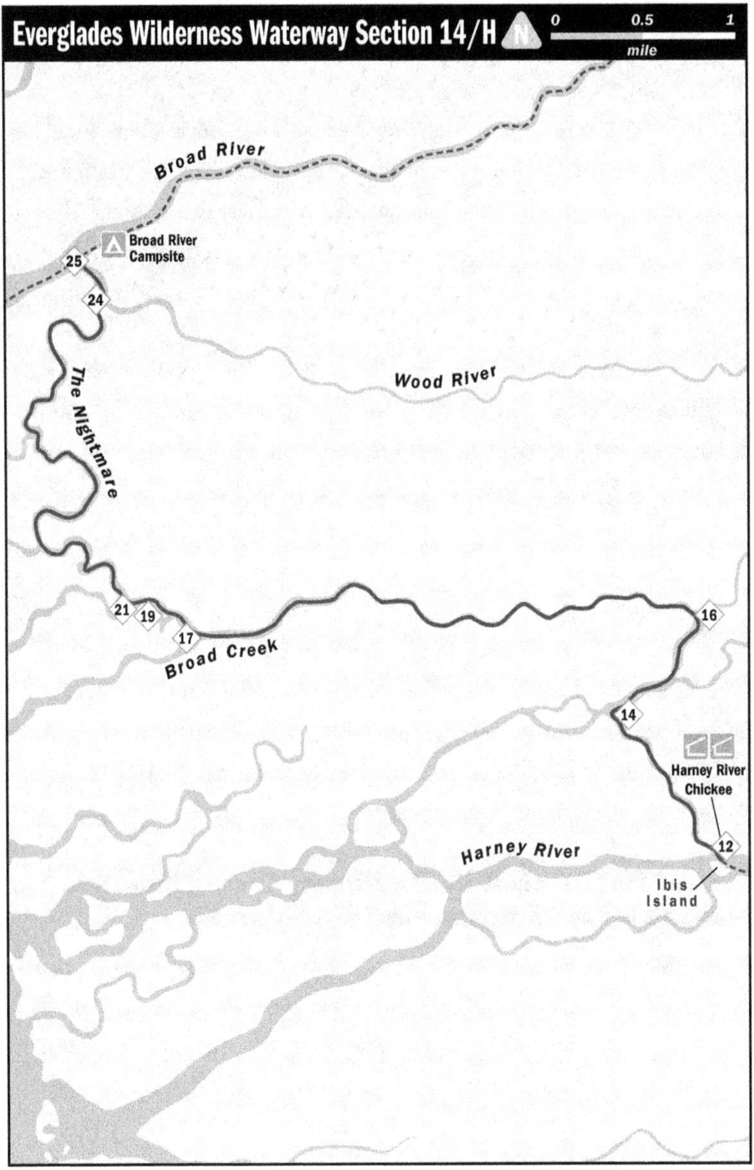
Everglades Wilderness Waterway Section 14/H
N
0
0.5
1
mile
Broad River
Broad River Campsite
25
24
Wood River
The Nightmare
21
19
17
Broad Creek
16
14
Harney River Chickee
12
Harney River
Ibis Island

lush with vegetation and bird life. If you are the morning's first traveler through this narrow, winding passage, you will have the honor of breaking all the spiderwebs.

There may be times when you will be uncertain if you are still on the main channel, so look for evidence of cut branches, which indicate that someone in the past may have worked to clear the passage. You won't get lost if you remember to keep right, keep right, keep right, except where markers indicate passages to the Gulf. Pass those by.

A little more than halfway through The Nightmare you will see marker 23, which indicates the first passage out to the Gulf. Later 21 and 19 mark the second, and then 17 indicates the junction of The Nightmare with Broad Creek. Turn left (east) into Broad Creek. (A right turn would take you out to the Gulf.)

The creek starts out as an easier paddle than The Nightmare, but it soon narrows into a passage equally twisting and challenging. At least you won't have to worry here about being stranded at low tides. The creek turns southwesterly at marker 16, and then southeasterly at marker 14, where the channel opens a bit. You will reach the Harney River and the Harney River Chickee at marker 12. The marker is nailed to the chickee.

SOUTH TO NORTH: Harney River Chickee to Broad River Campsite via The Nightmare

To paddle Broad Creek and The Nightmare, turn northwest into the channel on the back side of the Harney River Chickee. Follow this channel and turn right (northeast) at marker 14. Unlike paddling The Nightmare, you can paddle Broad Creek at any tide, but take care not to hit The Nightmare at low tide because it will be impassable.

At marker 16 turn left (west), following Broad Creek to marker 17, which marks the entrance to The Nightmare. If you are near low tide at this point, you could decide to continue west past marker 17 to the Gulf, and then head north up the Gulf Coast to the Broad River, rather than risk getting stuck.

To paddle The Nightmare, take the right (northwest) channel at marker 17. The Nightmare is a narrow, twisting passage that winds in a northerly direction. It has earned its name for the work you will have to do ducking under and passing over mangrove branches and roots, but the beauty of the foliage and company of waterbirds will be your reward.

There may be times when you will be uncertain if you are still on the main channel, especially when water is high and the channel has spread into the mangroves. You can look for weathered ends of cut branches, which indicate that at some time, someone cleared the passage. Generally, just keep left, keep left, keep left, bypassing markers 19, 21, and 23, which mark passages to the Gulf. Continue to marker 24 at The Nightmare's end at the Wood River. Turn left (north) and you will arrive quickly at marker 25 and the Broad River.

Turn right (northeast) up the Broad, and the Broad River Campsite will soon appear on your right.

SECTION 15/G

HARNEY RIVER CHICKEE/MARKER 9 OR CANEPATCH CAMPSITE

Harney River Chickee (marker 12): N25° 25.953' W81° 05.464'
Marker 9: N25° 24.903' W81° 00.441'
Canepatch Campsite: N25° 25.317' W80° 56.619'
Estimated paddling distance, Harney River Chickee/marker 9: 5.5 miles
Estimated paddling distance, Harney River Chickee/Canepatch Campsite: 9.5 miles

NORTH TO SOUTH: Harney River Chickee to Marker 9 or Canepatch Campsite

Leave the Harney River Chickee and turn left, traveling east along the Harney River. Navigating this river is relatively easy as you follow the course of the river for approximately 8 miles, but be aware that the Harney can be a challenge to paddle if the wind is out of the east and you face the headwind, the tide, and the river's current. If the wind is from the west, however, the Harney is a breeze—but then the Shark River can be challenging.

You will soon see marker 11, which indicates where the North Harney River branches off to the left. Pass marker 11 and continue straight along the main course of the Harney. You will see several water-monitoring stations along the Harney's banks.

About 5 miles after you leave the Harney River Chickee, you will come to marker 9 indicating the western end of Tarpon Bay. Turn right (south) onto the Shark River.

If you plan to stay at Canepatch Campsite, enter Tarpon Bay rather than turning south at marker 9. Paddle east across Tarpon Bay until it divides at a large island. Take the right (south) branch of the bay until you see ahead of you a peninsula that points toward you from the eastern end of the bay. Go left of the peninsula into Avocado Creek, very narrow and clear. Paddle a little over 1 mile up this creek until you come to a small lagoon. Canepatch

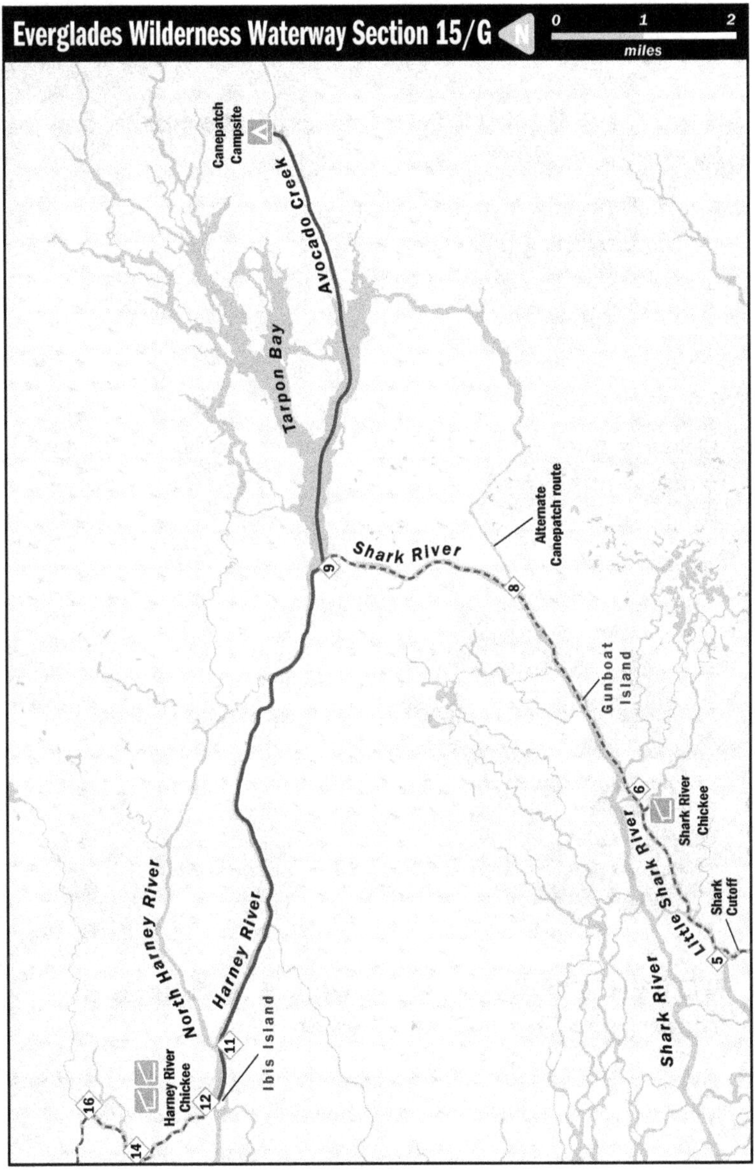
Everglades Wilderness Waterway Section 15/G
N
0
1
2
miles
Canepatch Campsite
Avocado Creek
Tarpon Bay
Shark River
Alternate Canepatch route
9
8
Gunboat Island
6
Shark River Chickee
Shark River
Little Shark River
Shark Cutoff
5
North Harney River
Harney River
11
12
Ibis Island
Harney River Chickee
16
14

Campsite sits on the left. In the morning, retrace your route to marker 9 and head south into the Shark River.

SOUTH TO NORTH: Canepatch Campsite or Marker 9 to Harney River Chickee

If you stayed at Canepatch Campsite, retrace your path in the morning, traveling west along Avocado Creek and Tarpon Bay to marker 9.

At marker 9 continue west along the Harney River for approximately 5.5 miles. Do not take the channels that branch off to the right, but stay in the main body of the Harney. You will finally see marker 11 and, 0.5 mile farther, marker 12 attached to the Harney River Chickee. Be sure to pass to the right of Ibis Island in the middle of the Harney, or you might miss the chickee and marker 12.

SECTION 16/F

MARKER 9 OR CANEPATCH CAMPSITE/ SHARK RIVER CHICKEE

Marker 9: N25° 24.903' W81° 00.441'
Canepatch Campsite: N25° 25.317' W80° 56.619'
Shark River Chickee: N25° 22.180' W81° 02.804'
Estimated paddling distance, marker 9/Shark River Chickee: 4.5 miles
Estimated paddling distance, Canepatch Campsite/Shark River Chickee: 8.5 miles

NORTH TO SOUTH: Marker 9 or Canepatch Campsite to Shark River Chickee

From marker 9, paddle south to pass marker 8 on your left, and continue on to Gunboat Island in the middle of Shark River (see page 260). The island's shape suggests a boat heading upriver—thus its name. You can paddle either side of it, depending on which side gives you relief from the wind if that has been a

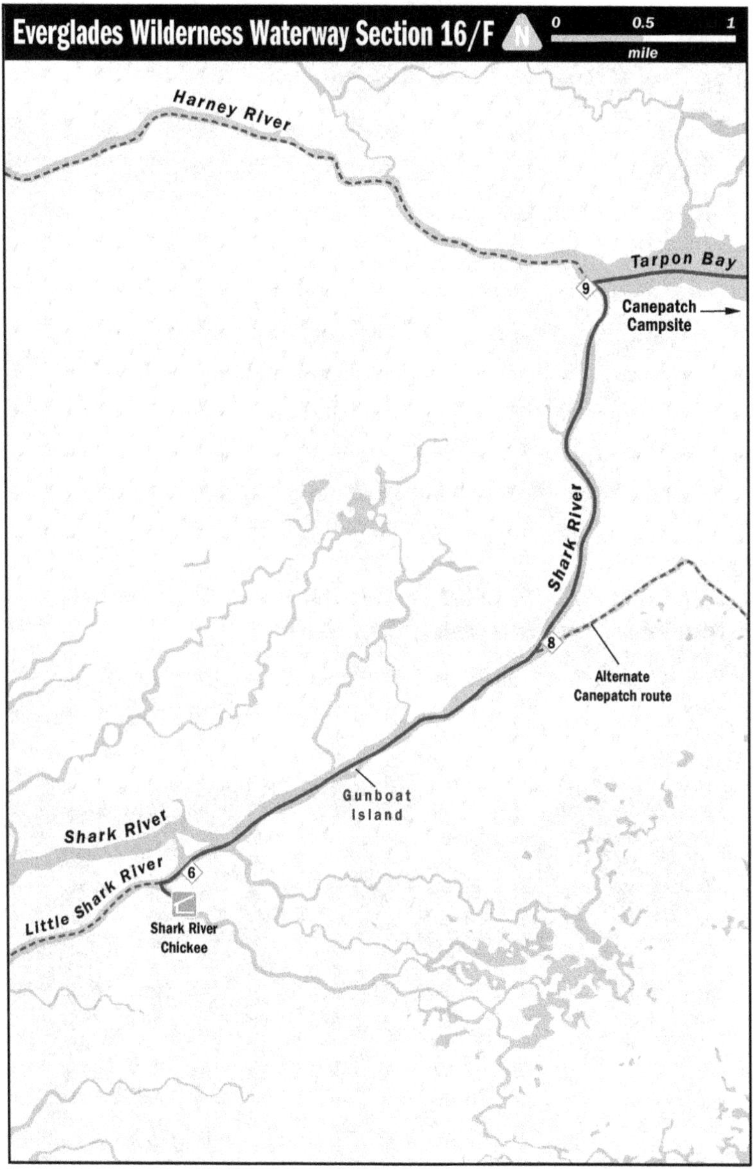
Everglades Wilderness Waterway Section 16/F
N
0
0.5
1
mile
Harney River
Tarpon Bay
9
Canepatch Campsite
Shark River
8
Alternate Canepatch route
Gunboat Island
Shark River
Little Shark River
6
Shark River Chickee

problem. In another 1.5 miles the main branch of the Shark breaks off to the right, but stay to the left on the Little Shark River, passing marker 6.

Continue down the Little Shark a short way to the first side channel that branches to the left. Take this channel to the Shark River Chickee, which is quickly visible.

If you are traveling from Canepatch Campsite, paddle west back along Avocado Creek into Tarpon Bay and travel 2.5 miles across the bay to marker 9. Turn left (south) at marker 9 and paddle down the Shark River, passing marker 8 and Gunboat Island.

When the Shark River branches off to the right, continue straight down the Little Shark River. Pass marker 6 and take the next channel to the left. The Shark River Chickee lies just down this channel on the right shoreline.

SOUTH TO NORTH: Shark River Chickee to Marker 9 or Canepatch Campsite

When leaving the Shark River Chickee, rejoin the Little Shark River, turning right (northeast). Soon after marker 6, the Little

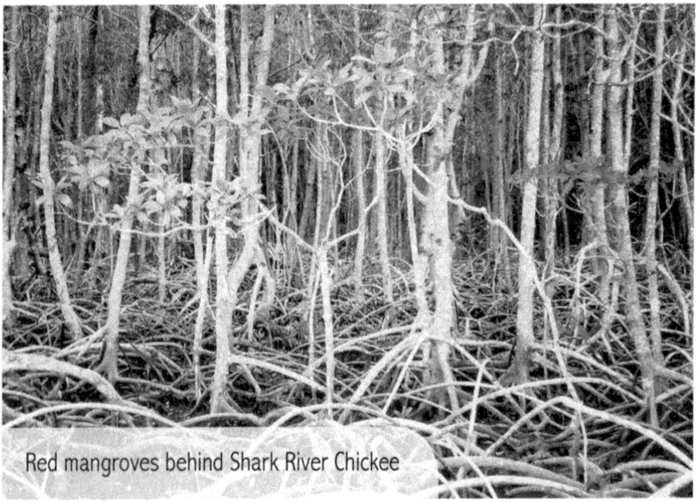

Red mangroves behind Shark River Chickee

Shark River joins the Shark River, which comes in on the left. You will be traveling in a northeasterly direction and will pass Gunboat Island and then, in a little more than 1 mile, marker 8, where the Shark River takes a more northerly turn to the left. You will pass water-monitoring stations as you continue to marker 9, where the Shark River meets the Harney River at Tarpon Bay.

As a northbound traveler, if you are heading to Canepatch Campsite to break up your journey before you paddle to marker 9, you may want to take the unnamed channel that branches to the right (northeast) at marker 8 (see Section 15/G map on page 99). This channel courses 1 mile northeast, turns right, and continues 1 mile southeast, then turns left (northeast, again) for a little more than a mile, and then left (north) for over another mile. You will enter Tarpon Bay close to the spot where Avocado Creek leads east to Canepatch. Check your charts. This route variation is not difficult to follow. Of course, you can always continue on the Shark directly to marker 9 and then turn right into Tarpon Bay and east to Avocado Creek and Canepatch Campsite.

SECTION 17/E

SHARK RIVER CHICKEE/OYSTER BAY CHICKEE

Shark River Chickee: N25° 22.180' W81° 02.804'
Oyster Bay Chickee: N25° 19.410' W81° 03.981'
Estimated paddling distance: 5 miles

NORTH TO SOUTH: Shark River Chickee to Oyster Bay Chickee

From Shark River Chickee, return to the main channel of the Little Shark River. Paddle left (southwest) to marker 5, where you turn left (south) into the Shark Cutoff. At marker 3 you enter the northeast end of Oyster Bay. Paddle in a southeasterly direction, watching for marker 2.

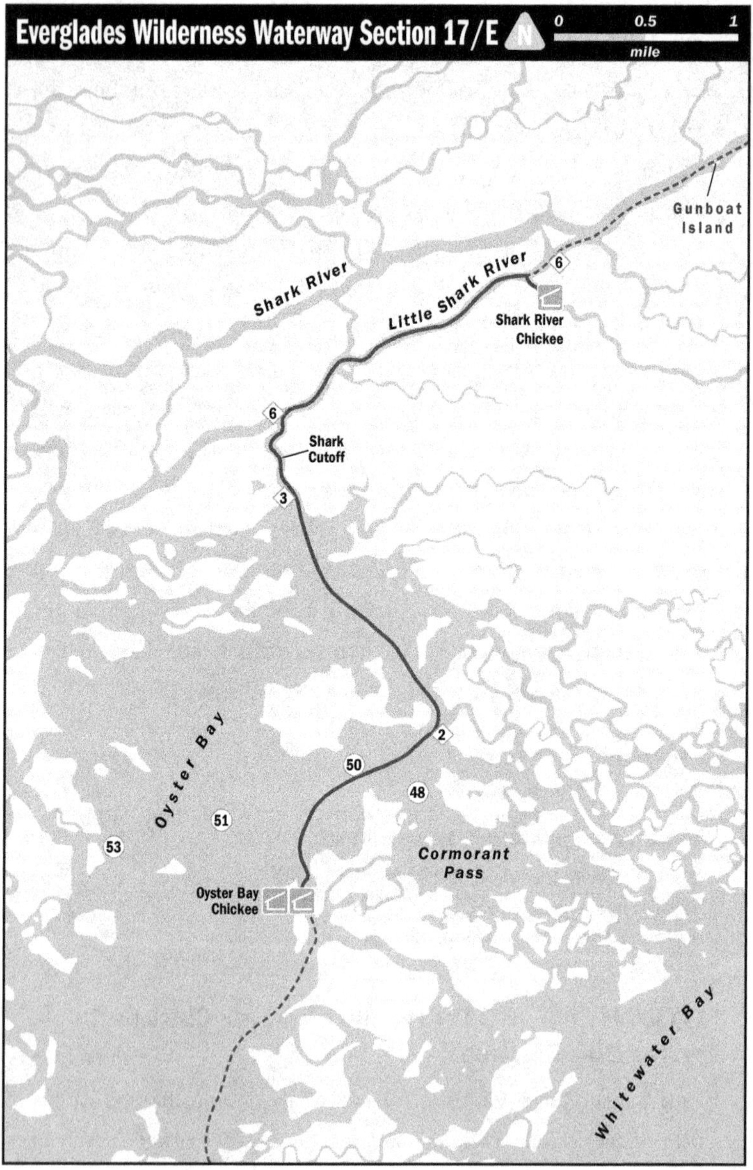
Everglades Wilderness Waterway Section 17/E
N
0
0.5
1
mile
Gunboat Island
6
Shark River
Little Shark River
Shark River Chickee
6
Shark Cutoff
3
2
50
48
Oyster Bay
51
53
Cormorant Pass
Oyster Bay Chickee
Whitewater Bay

The historical Wilderness Waterway crosses Whitewater Bay at this point. We do not recommend this route, as it involves crossing approximately 12 miles of open water, where you will have to deal with motorboaters and the wind and waves. Whitewater Bay has earned its name.

Instead, head southwest from Wilderness Waterway marker 2 into Oyster Bay and pass between USCG marker 48 to the east and USCG marker 50 to the west. Tucked in behind mangroves, Oyster Bay Chickee sits in a cove on the *west* side of the island that lies 0.5 mile directly south of USCG marker 50. This chickee is hard to spot as it is hidden in a cluster of islands and not clearly marked on the NOAA charts or the Waterproof Charts. Look for the *arrow* on the NOAA chart 11433 to help locate this chickee.

SOUTH TO NORTH: Oyster Bay Chickee to Shark River Chickee

When leaving Oyster Bay Chickee, travel 0.5 mile farther north and you will see the USCG markers that indicate the route from the Gulf of Mexico east to Whitewater Bay. Pass between USCG marker 48 to your right (east) and USCG marker 50 to your left (west). Particularly on weekends, motorboaters follow these markers to and from Whitewater Bay.

Directly north of USCG marker 48 is Wilderness Waterway marker 2. Paddle northeast through this channel, and then maintain a northwest course as you cross the northern portion of Oyster Bay. Marker 3 indicates the entrance to the Shark River Cutoff.

Follow the cutoff until it merges with the Little Shark River at marker 5. Turn right (northeast) into the Little Shark. Continuing up the river you will pass a stream that crosses the Little Shark. Continue on the Little Shark until the *second* stream. Turning right (southeast) onto this channel, you will see the Shark River Chickee immediately on your right.

SECTION 18/D

OYSTER BAY CHICKEE/JOE RIVER CHICKEE

Oyster Bay Chickee: N25° 19.410' W81° 03.981'
Joe River Chickee: N25° 16.789' W81° 03.942'
Estimated paddling distance: 4 miles

NORTH TO SOUTH: Oyster Bay Chickee to Joe River Chickee

Paddle south down Oyster Bay, and keep heading south until you reach the southern end of this bay. Because this section is not identified by Wilderness Waterway markers, you will need to rely on your compass and charts. Conditions with winds and waves can pose obstacles in this section of your thru-paddle. If necessary, hug the shoreline to get some relief behind the islands. Generally, you're more likely to get a calm paddle in the morning rather than later in the day.

At the south end of Oyster Bay, Mud Bay lies to the southwest and the Joe River to the southeast. Look for the MANATEE ZONE sign on your left, marking the entrance to the Joe River. Shortly, you will see the Joe River Chickee in a cove to your left (north).

SOUTH TO NORTH: Joe River Chickee to Oyster Bay Chickee

Paddle out of the Joe River Chickee's little cove, turning right and rejoining the Joe River. Very soon at the mouth of the Joe River, which is marked by a MANATEE ZONE sign, Mud Bay opens to your left (southwest) and the expanse of Oyster Bay to your right (north).

In this unmarked area with many islands, use your compass and navigational charts to travel north up Oyster Bay and, if

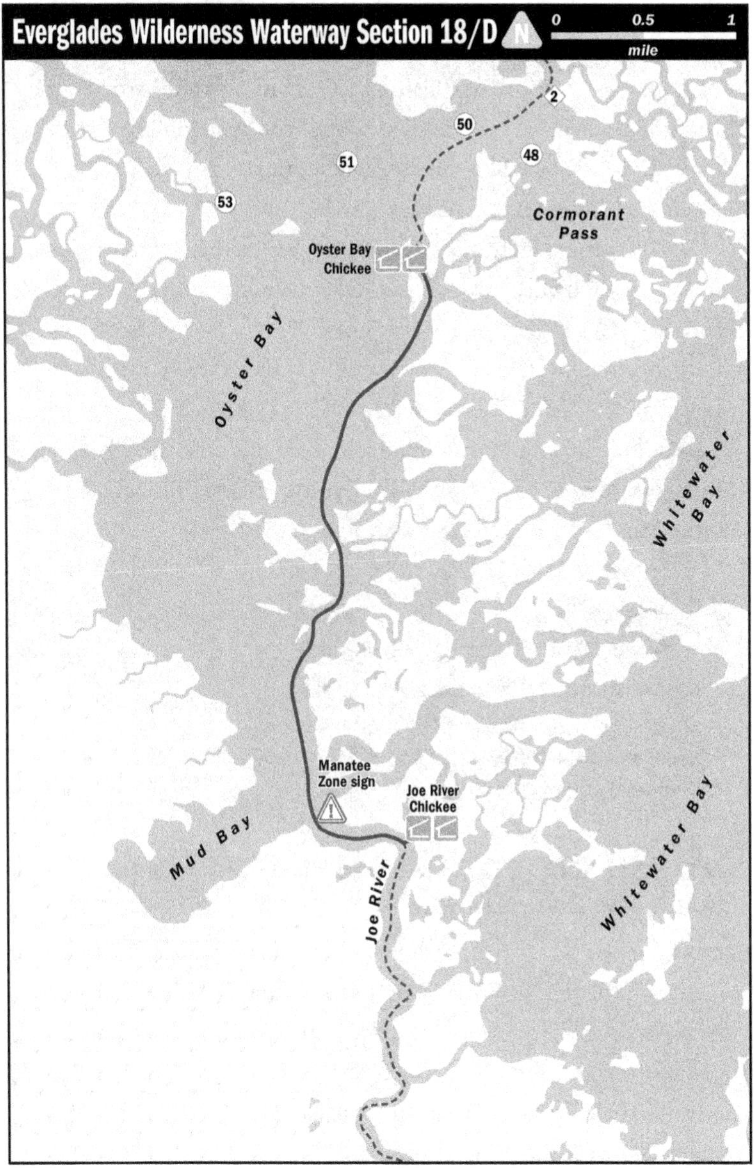
Everglades Wilderness Waterway Section 18/D
N
0
0.5
1
mile
2
50
48
51
53
Cormorant Pass
Oyster Bay Chickee
Oyster Bay
Whitewater Bay
Manatee Zone sign
Joe River Chickee
Mud Bay
Joe River
Whitewater Bay

the winds and waves are strong, keep close to the shore to your right, getting some protection in the lee of the islands.

A note about mangroves: It's hard to differentiate one mangrove island from another when you're paddling because they often look just like the shoreline until you get close to them. (Also see "Mangrove," on page 253.)

Approximately 3.5 miles north on Oyster Bay on the right, Oyster Bay Chickee is somewhat hidden among mangrove islands, and the NOAA charts and Waterproof Charts are a bit confusing as to its location. Note the location arrow on the NOAA Whitewater Bay Chart 11433. *Note:* If you reach USCG marker 50, you have passed the chickee. Turn around and head 0.5 mile directly south from the marker to the first island you come to. The chickee is tucked in a cove on the western side of that island.

SECTION 19/C

JOE RIVER CHICKEE/SOUTH JOE RIVER CHICKEE

Joe River Chickee: N25° 16.789' W81° 03.942'
South Joe River Chickee: N25° 13.320' W81° 00.641'
Estimated paddling distance: 6.5 miles

NORTH TO SOUTH: Joe River Chickee to South Joe River Chickee

From the Joe River Chickee, exit the cove and turn left, continuing down the Joe River traveling south-southeast. The Joe River is wide, and there is a good chance that you will pass motorboaters, so stay to the right. All of the cutoffs you encounter will be to the left (north); these are channels that connect the Joe River to Whitewater Bay. The potential difficulty of paddling this stretch is that you may encounter a headwind and/or experience strong cross-currents and winds from Whitewater Bay as you pass the channels.

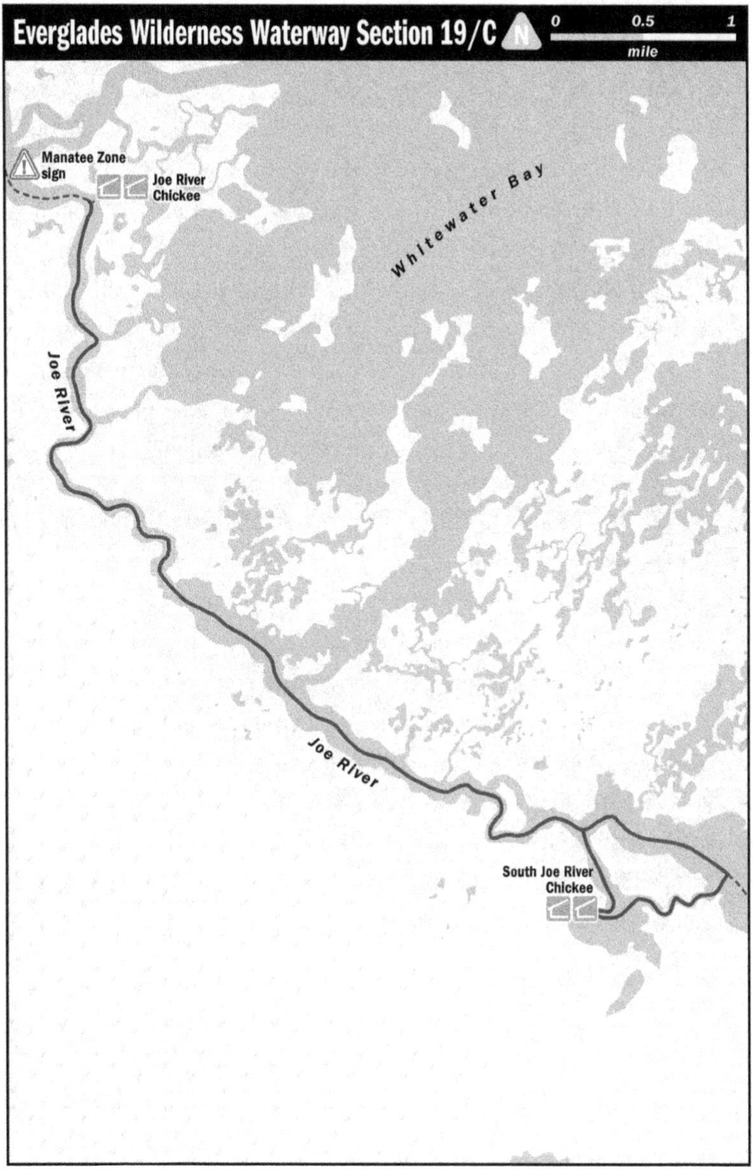
Everglades Wilderness Waterway Section 19/C
N
0
0.5
1
mile
Manatee Zone sign
Joe River Chickee
Whitewater Bay
Joe River
Joe River
South Joe River Chickee

It is approximately 6.5 miles between the Joe River Chickee and the South Joe River Chickee. The only bit of tricky navigation before you reach the South Joe River Chickee is finding the entrance to the bay where the chickee is located. Watch for a channel that branches off to the right (south) and takes you behind a large mangrove island to the bay. Once inside the bay, you will see the chickee in the northwest corner.

If you miss the first channel, take the next right (south) turn. If you see a MANATEE ZONE sign on the left (north) side of the Joe, you have gone a bit too far. Turn back and take the first channel to the left. (Always keep in mind, however, that signs appear and disappear out here. They must not be your only indicators.)

SOUTH TO NORTH: South Joe River Chickee to Joe River Chickee

Leave the South Joe River Chickee via the left (northwest) channel to rejoin the Joe River. Turn left (northwest) and continue up the Joe, traveling approximately 6 miles before coming to the Joe River Chickee. Navigating is easy because all of the cutoffs—channels leading to Whitewater Bay—will be to the right (north). Nevertheless, depending on conditions, this can be a challenging paddle with high winds and crosscurrents at the inlets.

The Joe River Chickee is a double chickee, visible from the Joe, in a little cove on the right (north) side of the river.

SECTION 20/B

SOUTH JOE RIVER CHICKEE/TARPON CREEK

South Joe River Chickee: N25° 13.320' W81° 00.641'
Tarpon Creek: N25° 12.708' W80° 55.857'
Estimated paddling distance: 6.5 miles

NORTH TO SOUTH: South Joe River Chickee to Tarpon Creek

Return to the Joe River, turn right, and continue paddling southeast. When the Joe River turns east, it widens progressively until you reach the entrance to Tarpon Creek. If you paddle on a windy day, take care, especially if the wind is against you, as this is open water. We once had to paddle this section on a day with a small-craft advisory. It was a serious challenge. Watch for USCG marker 10 at the entrance to Tarpon Creek.

SOUTH TO NORTH: Tarpon Creek to South Joe River Chickee

At USCG marker 10, Tarpon Creek opens onto the Joe River to the left (west) and Whitewater Bay to the north.

Navigational charts show the Everglades Wilderness Waterway crossing the open waters of Whitewater Bay. We do not recommend paddling that route, which involves crossing approximately 12 miles of open water, where you will have to deal with motorboaters and often rough waters. The Seminole name *wiwahatki* combines *wiwa*, meaning "water," with *hatki*, meaning "white." The word *whitewater* aptly describes this often windy bay.

Instead, paddle directly west (left) from USCG marker 10 onto the Joe River, which is wide at this point. This may be a difficult, wavy paddle if the wind is up and against you.

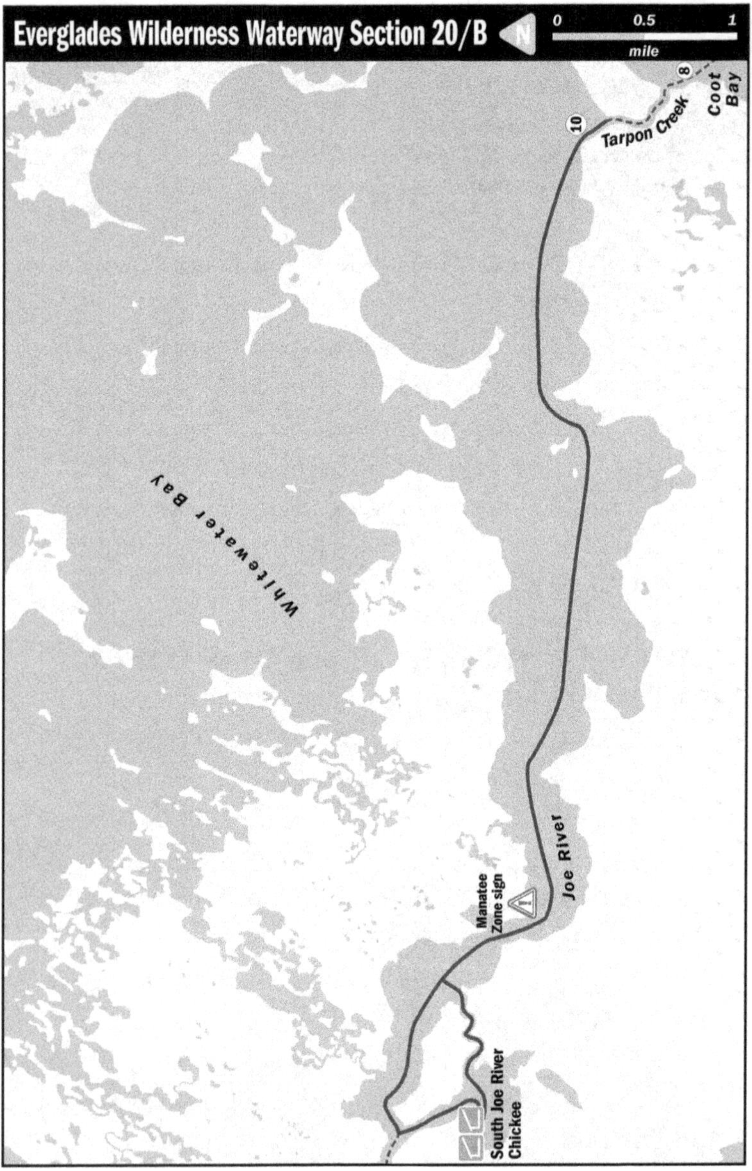
Everglades Wilderness Waterway Section 20/B
N
0
0.5
1
mile
Coot Bay
8
Tarpon Creek
10
Whitewater Bay
Joe River
Manatee Zone sign
South Joe River Chickee

Monitor your navigational chart as you paddle approximately 6 miles on the Joe River. Take the channel that cuts off to the left (west) and leads behind a large mangrove island to the South Joe River Chickee. A MANATEE ZONE sign on the right (northern) shore of the Joe River indicates that your channel will shortly appear on your left. If you miss this channel, look for the next. You will loop behind the same mangrove island. The South Joe River Chickee is positioned on the northwest side of the small bay behind the island. You cannot see the chickee until you are in the bay.

SECTION 21/A

TARPON CREEK/FLAMINGO

Tarpon Creek: N25° 12.708' W80° 55.857'
Flamingo: N25° 08.624' W80° 55.354'
Estimated paddling distance: 5 miles

NORTH TO SOUTH: Tarpon Creek to Flamingo

Watch for USCG marker 10 at the entrance to Tarpon Creek. Paddle south down the creek to USCG marker 8, where the creek enters Coot Bay. USCG markers 6 to 3 lead southeast across the bay, and USCG markers 2 and 1 (a green floating barrel) indicate the entrance to the Buttonwood Canal (see page 246).

Continue south through the canal. You may pass motorboaters, possibly a park service tour boat, and paddlers who have rented canoes from the concessionaire in Flamingo. Use caution and keep to the right. When you see these boaters out for a couple of easy hours, you will feel a sense of satisfaction in having spent more than a week paddling deep in the Everglades wilderness.

The Buttonwood Canal is a slow, easy paddle after what you've accomplished. Enjoy it. Admire the air plants. Notice

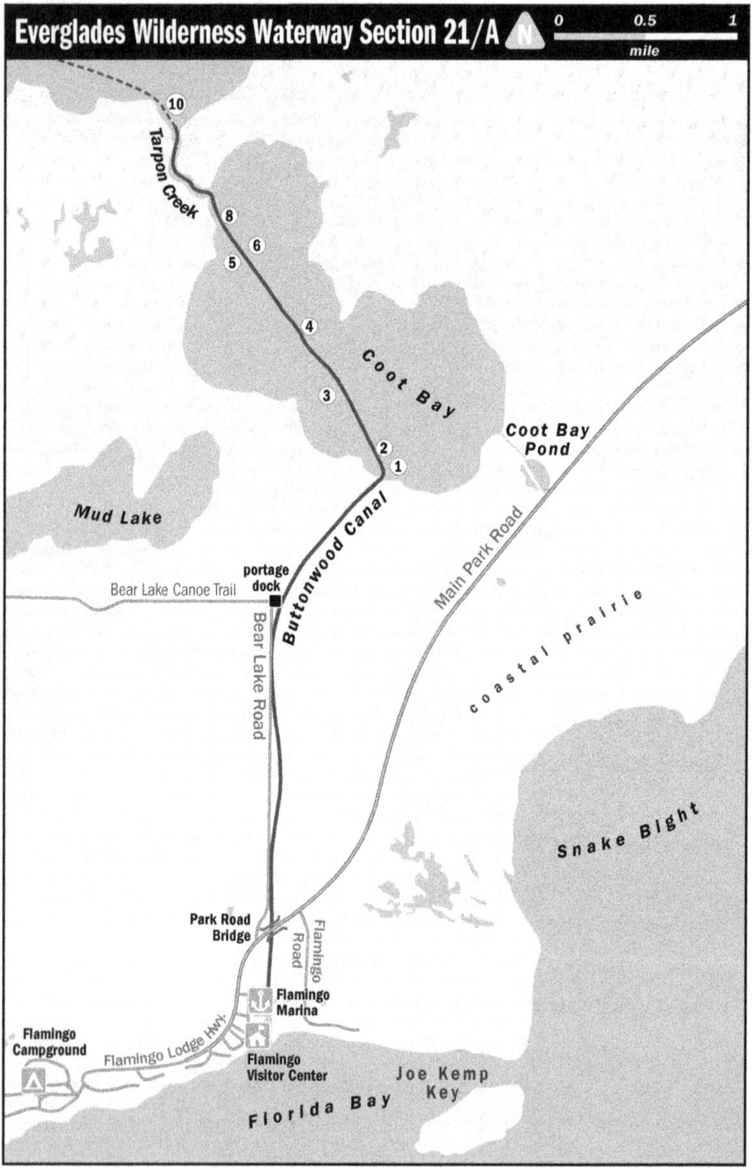
Everglades Wilderness Waterway Section 21/A
N
0
0.5
1
mile
10
Tarpon Creek
8
6
5
4
3
Coot Bay
2
1
Coot Bay Pond
Mud Lake
Buttonwood Canal
Main Park Road
portage dock
Bear Lake Canoe Trail
Bear Lake Road
coastal prairie
Snake Bight
Park Road Bridge
Flamingo Road
Flamingo Marina
Flamingo Campground
Flamingo Lodge Hwy.
Flamingo Visitor Center
Joe Kemp Key
Florida Bay

the limestone to your right, the bedrock of the Everglades. Just before the Park Road Bridge, look for one of the resident American crocodiles that may be sunning on the bank to your right. (See more on limestone, on page 253, and the American crocodile, on page 245.)

After paddling under the bridge, take out your boat at the Flamingo marina docks, the final point of your journey along the Everglades Wilderness Waterway.

SOUTH TO NORTH: Flamingo to Tarpon Creek

Launching at Flamingo, you will have the convenience of floating docks to facilitate loading. Be careful if you use the boat ramp, as it is slippery with algae.

As you leave the launch, head north, straight up the Buttonwood Canal. Stay to the right, as you may pass motorboaters, possibly a park service tour boat, and paddlers who have rented their boats from the Flamingo concessionaire. On your left, you will see limestone formations and possibly a resident American crocodile sunning itself on the left bank. (See more on limestone, on page 253, and the American crocodile, on page 245.)

When you exit the Buttonwood Canal onto Coot Bay you will see USCG marker 1 painted on a green floating barrel, as well as USCG marker 2. Paddle northwest across Coot Bay following USCG markers 3–6 to marker 8, which, along with a NO WAKE/MANATEE ZONE sign, marks the entrance to Tarpon Creek.

Paddle Tarpon Creek north to USCG marker 10, where the creek opens onto the Joe River to the left (west) and Whitewater Bay to the north.

MAP 22: The Historical Route

At the southern end of the original 100-mile Wilderness Waterway route, northbound paddlers are directed to cross Whitewater

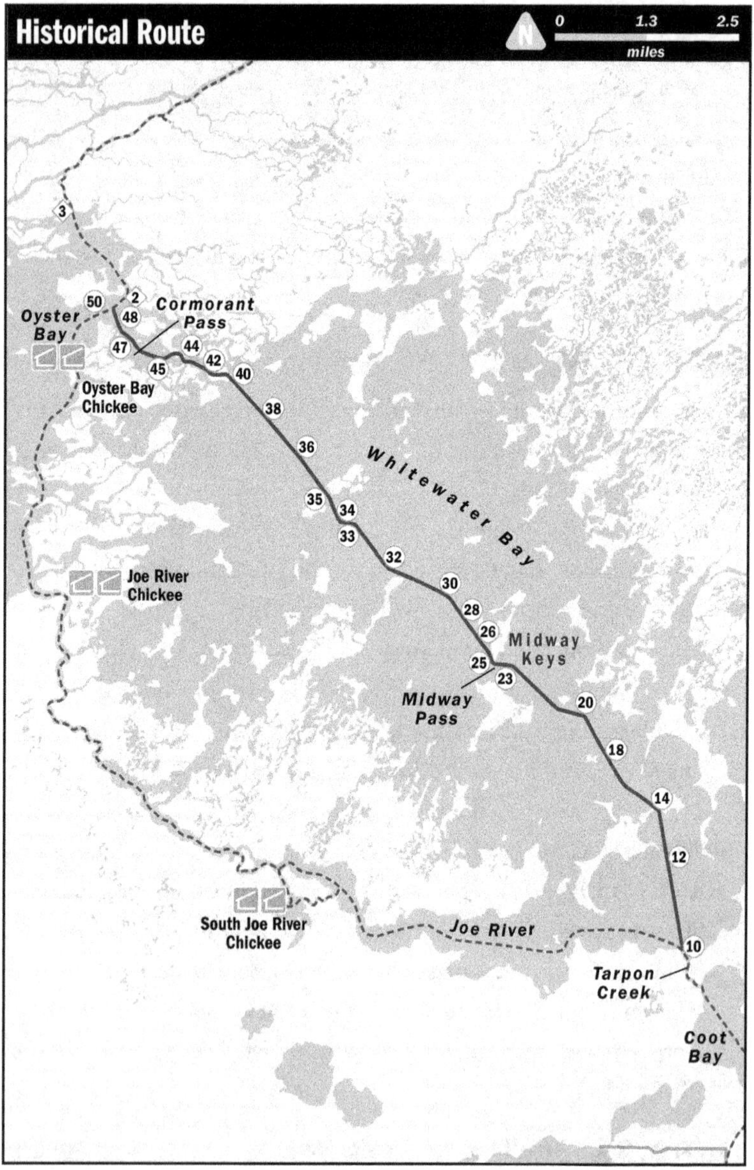
Historical Route
0
1.3
2.5
miles
3
2
50
48
Cormorant
Pass
Oyster
Bay
47
44
42
45
40
Oyster Bay
Chickee
38
36
Whitewater Bay
35
34
33
32
Joe River
Chickee
30
28
26
Midway
Keys
25
23
Midway
Pass
20
18
14
12
South Joe River
Chickee
Joe River
10
Tarpon
Creek
Coot
Bay

Bay between USCG markers numbered from 10 to 48 to Wilderness Waterway marker 2. For southbound paddlers, it's between USCG markers numbered from 48 to 10. The NOAA charts and Waterproof Charts, as well as the Truesdell guidebook, show this route. However, paddling across Whitewater Bay is *not* recommended: it involves crossing approximately 12 miles of wide and open water where the winds and waves can be hazardous and conditions can change rapidly. A safer trip that avoids Whitewater Bay, the Joe River route, is described in the text and maps for sections 18/D–20/B in this guidebook.

The Joe River and South Joe River chickees were constructed and placed with paddlers in mind (though they are also open to motorboaters). The intent was to locate the sites off the more heavily traveled route and provide some seclusion. We are including a map of the original route here for reference.

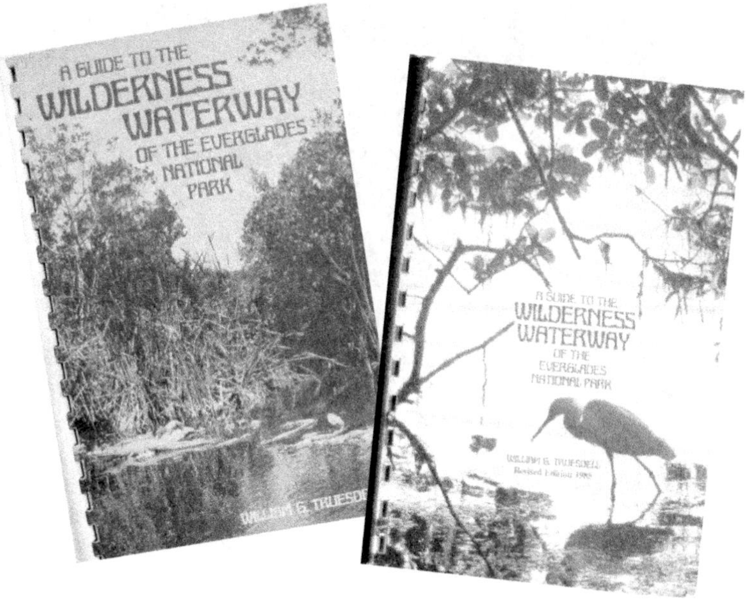

The first and second editions of William G. Truesdell's guidebook

Paddler on Halfway Creek

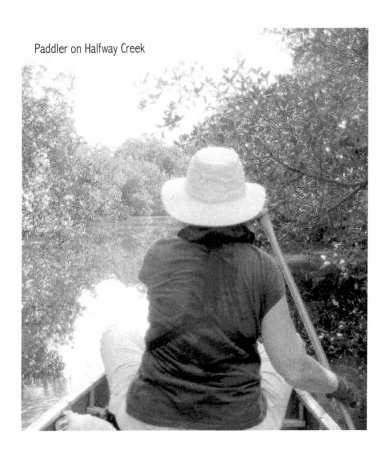

Part Two:

North Everglades Day & Overnight Paddles

When you don't have the time or inclination to negotiate the full Everglades Wilderness Waterway, you can still enjoy this extraordinary maritime environment as only a paddler can. In this section, we describe five day trips and three overnight excursions that offer diverse experiences for a range of paddling skills.

All eight of these North Everglades trips originate from—and end in—Everglades City at the Gulf Coast Visitor Center, the westernmost of the Everglades visitor centers.

Each paddle included here is a loop or an out-and-back, so no shuttles are required. Canoe and kayak rentals are available from the concessionaire at the Gulf Coast VC, as well as from outfitters in Everglades City and at nearby Chokoloskee Island. (See Appendix 2, Launch Sites, on page 269; Appendix 3, Outfitters, Suppliers, & Canoe/Kayak Rentals, on page 275; and Appendix 4, Resource Overview, on page 278.)

PLAN AHEAD

On these paddles, you won't be on a 10-day, 99-mile Wilderness Waterway section-by-section expedition like the one described in Part One. But please don't let planning take a backseat.

Read the "Trip Preparation" section, on page 32, and modify your supplies for a day trip or an overnight. If you are paddling in the summer months, consult Part Four, Summer Paddling, on page 201, as well.

THE NONNEGOTIABLE BASICS

We cannot overemphasize the importance of always carrying enough water (1 gallon per person per day), and don't forget snacks, insect repellent, sunscreen, lip balm, a hat, and sunglasses. Check weather predictions and tide tables.

RESERVATIONS

If you plan to camp in the backcountry, you must make reservations at either the Gulf Coast VC or the Flamingo VC—in person—within 24 hours of your launch.

DIRECTIONS

To get to the put-in at the Gulf Coast VC from the west (Naples), take I-75 east (Alligator Alley) through the first toll booth to Exit 80, FL 29 south. Travel approximately 20 miles south into Everglades City until you have to turn right. Enter the traffic circle and take the last exit from the circle. Continue straight until you come to Everglades National Park on your right. To access the marinas on Chokoloskee Island, continue 2 miles farther south, crossing the Chokoloskee Bridge and following the causeway onto the island.

From Miami, travel west on US 41 (the Tamiami Trail) for 62 miles and turn left onto FL 29 south. Travel approximately 3 miles into Everglades City. Follow FL 29 until you enter the traffic circle, and take the last exit from the circle. Continue straight until you come to Everglades National Park on your right. To access the marinas on Chokoloskee Island, continue 2 miles farther south, crossing the Chokoloskee Bridge and following the causeway onto the island.

DAY PADDLES—EVERGLADES CITY AREA

HALFWAY CREEK/TURNER RIVER LOOP

HALFWAY CREEK/TURNER RIVER LOOP

Distance: 11-mile loop

Paddle Time: 6 hours

Hazards: Muddy launch at low tide; strong tidal flow under Chokoloskee Bridge and in Turner River; heavy seasonal powerboat traffic in Chokoloskee Causeway Canal and on Turner River; mosquitoes in the mangrove tunnels in the rainy season

Gulf Coast VC: N25° 50.730' W81° 23.234'

Chokoloskee Bridge: N25° 50.381' W81° 22.884'

Plantation Island: N25° 50.619' W81° 22.419'

Fork in stream: N25° 50.995' W81° 21.254'

Turner Lake: N25° 50.902' W81° 20.001'

Turner River: N25° 49.921' W81° 20.302'

Shell mounds: N25° 49.618' W81° 20.535'

Maps & Charts: USGS Quadrangle *Chokoloskee, FL* 7.5-minute*; NOAA Chart 11430; Waterproof Chart 40E; a trip map may be available from the Gulf Coast VC, or download one from **nps.gov/ever/planyourvisit.** (*The short beginning and ending sections included in *Everglades City, FL* 7.5-minute are not necessary if this guidebook is followed.)

▶ **Description** Paddling this loop is a fine way to explore a variety of ecosystems in a one-day trip. You will pass through mangrove tunnels, narrow creeks, and broader rivers; visit a lake in the backcountry; and skirt the edge of Chokoloskee Bay. The route also takes you past sites of Everglades human history—the former pioneer settlement at Plantation Key and the Native American Calusa shell mounds tucked into the mangrove shores of the Turner River.

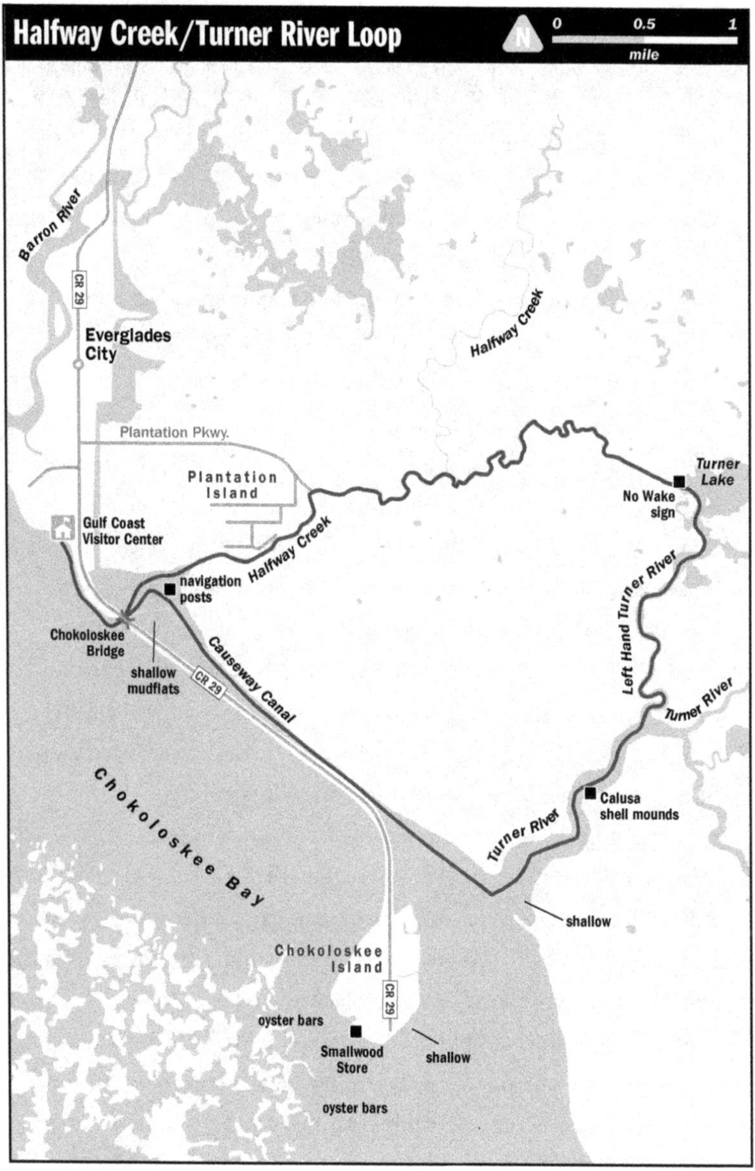
Halfway Creek/Turner River Loop
N
0
0.5
1
mile
Barron River
CR 29
Everglades City
Plantation Pkwy.
Plantation Island
Gulf Coast Visitor Center
Halfway Creek
Halfway Creek
Turner Lake
No Wake sign
Left Hand Turner River
Turner River
navigation posts
Chokoloskee Bridge
shallow mudflats
CR 29
Causeway Canal
Calusa shell mounds
Turner River
Chokoloskee Bay
shallow
Chokoloskee Island
CR 29
oyster bars
Smallwood Store
shallow
oyster bars

▶ **Route** Launch at the Gulf Coast VC and head left (south) following the shoreline to the Chokoloskee Bridge. Try to launch on a rising tide, which will help you as you turn left (east) and pass under the bridge. Continue straight (east) into Halfway Creek, following the wooden posts to avoid mudflats if the tide is low. (Do not turn left into the canal leading to the Barron River or right into the Chokoloskee Causeway Canal.) You will see the houses of Plantation Island on your left as you enter the creek.

Halfway Creek was the site of one of the more flourishing pioneer settlements in the Chokoloskee Bay area. As many as 10–12 families lived on the banks of the creek in the 1890s and grew sugarcane, bananas, peppers, tomatoes, melons, and cabbages for the Key West–to–New York trade. Early pioneer Ted Smallwood reminisced, in Charlton Tebeau's *Florida's Last Frontier: The History of Collier County,* that the first general election (in which Grover Cleveland won the presidency) was held in 1892 at the Halfway Creek settlement, where a ballot box was brought over from Key West along with "all the poll tax receipts, a jug of licker, a box of cigars. All we had to do was vote." Today as you paddle up the creek, you will pass homes built on pilings to prevent damage from storm surge, with wide, screened porches and boat lifts.

About 1 mile up the creek you leave the homes behind and enter Everglades National Park. Halfway Creek narrows and is bordered by lush vegetation, including red mangroves with dangling aerial roots and massive black mangroves to your right (east), with their noticeably black bark and pencil-like pneumatophores poking out of the wet ground. The creek narrows and becomes a "green tunnel" with tidal flow and bends and turns. Paddle carefully through this section to avoid bumping into the mangroves when the current is strong. About 2 miles in, Halfway Creek forks to the left. Stay on the wider (right) channel and continue on the twisty waterway. You will pass two wider places on the route. Stay to the left side of these openings. After the second open area the creek straightens out and continues for about 0.5 mile into Turner Lake. A NO WAKE sign at this spot is a warning for boaters who are entering the creek from the lake.

As you enter the lake, pass an island immediately to your right, and after the island turn right (south) into Left Hand Turner River. Paddle in a southerly direction along this channel, watching for the ibis, snowy egrets, ospreys, and roseate spoonbills that often perch in mangroves along the river, and for the fish that are feeding in these waters. About 1.5 miles down the river, you will join the Turner River, which flows in from the left (east). Continue south, and stay alert for fishing boats and tour boats that use this channel.

You are paddling in a historical area. The Turner River (see page 263) got its name from a U.S. Army Seminole War scout in the 1860s who returned to settle on the river in 1871. But this is recent history when you compare it to that of the Calusa (see page 247), who lived in this area around 2,000 years ago. Understanding that the area was protected from storms by outlying islands, they built shell mounds along the river to create lands above the tide line. These settlements, both the pioneer and the earlier Calusa, have been overgrown by mangroves, but if you look closely at the south bank of the Turner River about 0.25 mile from Chokoloskee Bay, you can still see the shell mounds and evidence of early habitation.

When you reach Chokoloskee Bay, turn right (north) into the Chokoloskee Causeway Canal. Paddle 2 miles north through the channel, staying right if the water is low. At the Chokoloskee Bridge, turn left (west) and pass under the bridge, ideally on an outgoing tide. Once in Chokoloskee Bay turn right (north) and paddle 0.5 mile to your takeout at the Gulf Coast VC.

LOPEZ RIVER ROUTE

LOPEZ RIVER ROUTE

Distance: 15 miles round-trip
Paddle Time: 7 hours round-trip, depending on tides
Hazards: Muddy launch at low tide; heavy seasonal powerboat traffic; strong tidal flow
Gulf Coast VC: N25° 50.730' W81° 23.234'
Chokoloskee Bridge: N25° 50.381' W81° 22.884'
WW marker 127: N25° 47.320' W81° 20.201'
Lopez River Campsite: N25° 47.275' W81° 18.374'
Maps & Charts: USGS Quadrangles *Everglades City, FL* 7.5-minute, *Chokoloskee, FL* 7.5-minute; NOAA Nautical Chart 11430; Waterproof Chart 41

▶ **Description** The Lopez River Route allows you to explore both Chokoloskee Bay and the Lopez River, two waterways that were important to early pioneers. You will visit the homesite of one of those 1890s settlers, Spaniard Gregorio Lopez, and explore the remnants of his homestead structures on the Calusa shell mound where he lived.

This 15-mile day paddle can be divided by staying overnight at the Lopez River Campsite. Be sure to make the mandatory campsite reservations in person at the Gulf Coast VC within 24 hours of your launch.

Alternatively, you may choose to launch from one of the marinas at Chokoloskee (see Appendix 4, Resource Overview, on page 278), which will shorten your paddle to 10 miles round-trip.

Either way, pay attention to the tides as you plan. A higher tide helps you avoid a muddy launch from the visitor center. An

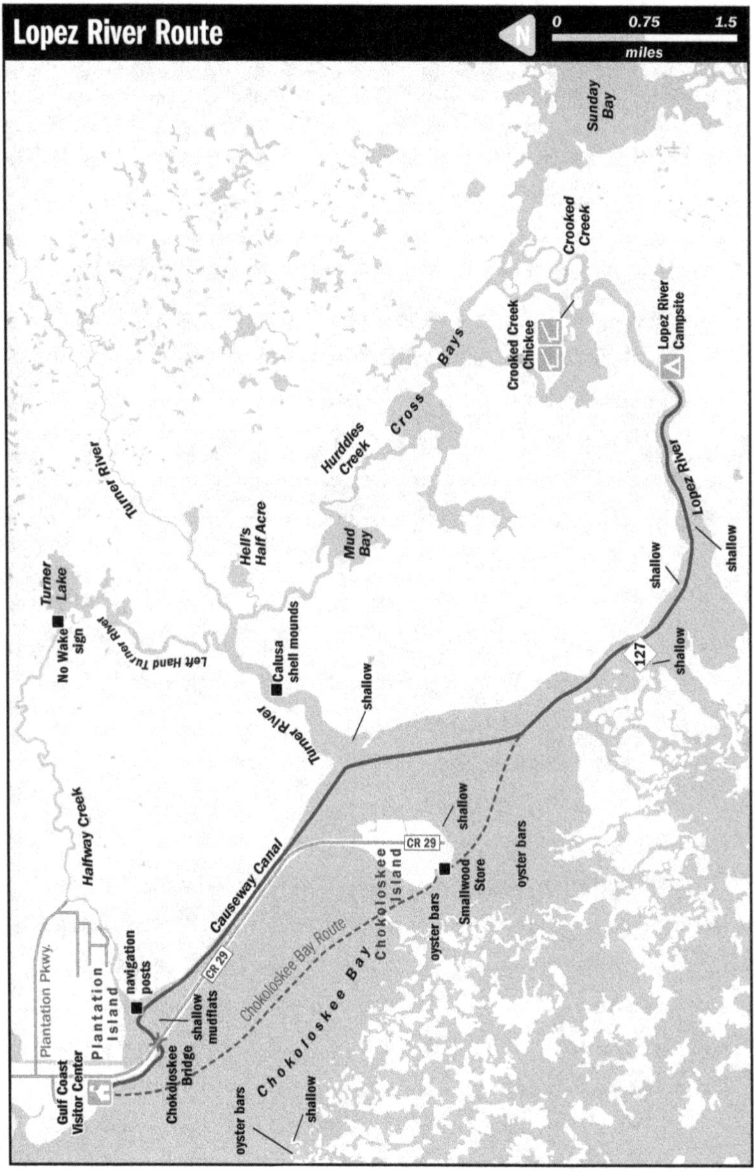
Lopez River Route
N
0
0.75
1.5
miles
Sunday Bay
Crooked Creek
Lopez River Campsite
Crooked Creek Chickee
Cross Bays
Hurddles Creek
Turner River
Hell's Half Acre
Mud Bay
Lopez River
shallow
shallow
Turner Lake
No Wake sign
Left Hand Turner River
Calusa shell mounds
shallow
127
shallow
Turner River
Halfway Creek
Causeway Canal
shallow
CR 29
Chokoloskee Island
Smallwood Store
oyster bars
Plantation Pkwy.
navigation posts
Plantation Island
CR 29
Chokoloskee Bay Route
oyster bars
shallow mudflats
Chokoloskee Bay
Gulf Coast Visitor Center
Chokoloskee Bridge
shallow
oyster bars

incoming tide makes the start of your journey—paddling under the Chokoloskee Bridge and up the Lopez River—much easier. An outgoing tide will aid in your paddle home.

▶ **Route** Launch your boat at the north side of the Gulf Coast VC in Everglades City. Paddle south along the shore to the Chokoloskee Bridge and turn left (east) under the bridge. Turn right (south) into the canal. If the water is shallow with a low tide, make this a wide right turn by following the small posts that lead to the left side of the channel, where the water is deeper. Do not be confused by the larger posts, which lead into Halfway Creek.

Paddle the 2-mile length of the canal, watching for green herons in the mangroves on the left, egrets and herons in the mud on the right, and mullet (see page 255) threatening to jump right into your boat. Stay alert for motorboaters.

When you leave the channel, travel southeast in Chokoloskee Bay, passing between Chokoloskee Island on your right (west) and Turner River on your left (east). Travel south down the bay, keeping the expanse of the bay to your right. Marker 127 indicates the mouth of the Lopez River. Numerous posts mark the deeper channel, if you find the water to be too shallow. Keep left and turn east into the Lopez River.

The Lopez River Campsite, marking Lopez's homestead, lies 2 miles up the river from marker 127. With its park service sign, concrete cistern, and modern privy, the Lopez site is easy to spot on the right bank of the river. Pull up to the shell beach and explore this historic destination. (See page 230 for more on the Lopez River Campsite.)

When you have finished exploring and possibly enjoying a picnic lunch among mangroves, buttonwoods, wild tamarind, and lush undergrowth, hopefully the tide will be falling, easing your paddle down the river, up the Causeway Canal, and under the

Chokoloskee Bridge as you return to the Gulf Coast VC for your takeout. If you are returning on a rising tide, consider paddling back on the west side of Chokoloskee Island rather than taking the canal, to avoid paddling against the tide under the bridge.

SANDFLY ISLAND

SANDFLY ISLAND

Distance: 4 miles round-trip

Paddle Time: 3 hours round-trip, depending on tides, plus 1 hour to walk the trail

Hazards: Muddy launch at low tide; heavy seasonal powerboat traffic; potential wind and waves in Chokoloskee Bay; strong tidal flow in Sandfly Pass; mosquitoes on Sandfly Island trail, especially in the summer

Gulf Coast VC: N25° 50.730' W81° 23.234'

USCG marker 2: N25° 49.803' W81° 23.515'

Sandfly Island: N25° 49.395' W81° 23.987'

Maps & Charts: USGS Quadrangle *Everglades City, FL* 7.5-minute; NOAA Nautical Chart 11430; Waterproof Chart 41; a trip map may be available from Gulf Coast VC, or download one from **nps.gov/ever/planyourvisit.**

▶ **Description** This trip takes you across the open waters of Chokoloskee Bay to historic Sandfly Island. In reality a horseshoe-shaped shell mound, the island was engineered more than 2,000 years ago by the Calusa mound builders. Evidence suggests that it was an active trading site where men and women would have been making shell tools, constructing fishing nets, and producing the rich material culture that archaeologists are discovering at Calusa sites.

The island became an animated place again from the 1870s through the early part of the 20th century. Names familiar in local lore and to area historians include former Seminole scout Captain Richard Turner, who lived at Sandfly until he moved

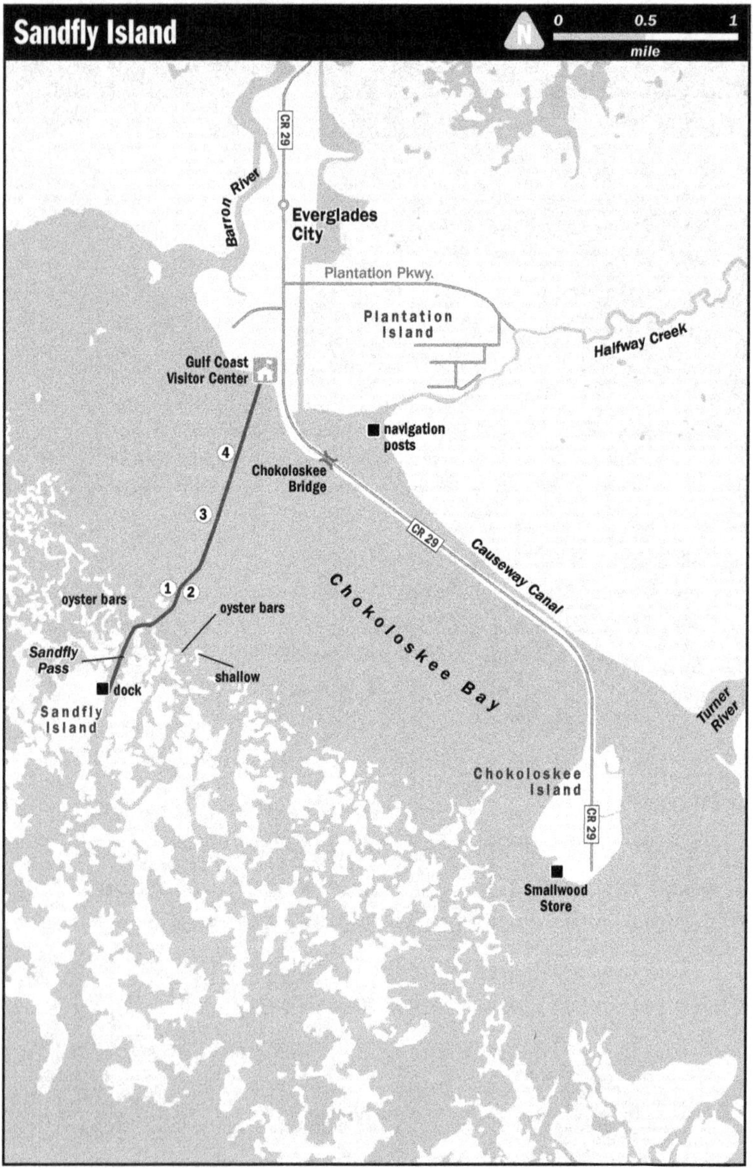
Sandfly Island
0
0.5
1
mile
N
CR 29
Barron River
Everglades City
Plantation Pkwy.
Plantation Island
Halfway Creek
Gulf Coast Visitor Center
navigation posts
4
Chokoloskee Bridge
3
CR 29
Causeway Canal
Chokoloskee Bay
1
2
oyster bars
oyster bars
Sandfly Pass
shallow
dock
Sandfly Island
Turner River
Chokoloskee Island
CR 29
Smallwood Store

to the Turner River and gave that river its name. In 1886 Joe Wiggins farmed and operated a small store here. Then there was Charley Boggess, who grew tomatoes, built a packing house, and boated his crop to market in Key West until 1923, when records show that he sold the island to Barron Collier. At about that time, Estelle Demere, who would later marry early resident and memoir writer Totch Brown, was born on a houseboat at Sandfly. Although the island is overgrown today, evidence of such pioneer habitation is seen in remains of a cistern and foundation blocks that lie on the 1-mile nature trail that encircles the island.

▶ **Route** To get closer to this history, launch at the north side of the Gulf Coast VC. On a clear day, you can spot the structures at Sandfly Island from the VC. The ideal time to launch is 2 hours before low tide so you can go out on the falling tide and catch the rising tide on your return, but this trip is possible at any tide.

Paddle southwest across Chokoloskee Bay, passing U.S. Coast Guard (USCG) markers 5 and 6 on your right (north). In the bay, you will see posts, one with reflective markings and the small notice U.S. DEPARTMENT OF THE INTERIOR BOUNDARY LINE, NATIONAL PARK SERVICE. Well before you arrive at Sandfly, you will spot the dock and the privy, but because of oyster beds, the markers lead you left of the channel that looks as if it would take you directly there. Look for USCG markers 1 and 2, which direct you into a deeper channel.

Once in Sandfly Pass, travel 0.5 mile to the dock on Sandfly Island. Pull up onto the small shell beach, as the dock can be slippery and difficult to access, and be sure to tie up to a mangrove to prevent your boat from floating away with the tide. The nature trail loop begins only steps from where you've tied up, with a sign illustrating a few facts about the history of the island.

Be sure to wear insect repellent and sturdy shoes if you intend to hike the 1-mile trail because it is thick with vegetation and, especially in the rainy season, can be thorny and overgrown in places. The trail loops back to the dock and beach where you began. Although rimmed by mangroves, the interior of the island is a profusion of wetland and upland vegetation—massive red-barked gumbo limbo trees (see page 251), a magnificent tamarind tree draped in Spanish moss, pungent-scented white stopper, pigeon plum, marlberry, white indigoberry, snowberry, coral bean, Jamaican caper, blue porterweed, wild lime, and wild coffee.

When you've enjoyed the nature trail, contemplated the island's rich history, and perhaps had a picnic on the dock, paddle back the way you came, ideally on a rising tide.

SANDFLY ISLAND LOOP

SANDFLY ISLAND LOOP

Distance: 4.5-mile loop

Paddle Time: 3 hours, depending on tides, plus 1 hour to hike the nature trail

Hazards: Muddy launch at low tide; heavy seasonal powerboat traffic; potential wind and waves in Chokoloskee Bay; strong tidal flow in Sandfly Pass; oyster beds at the south edge of Chokoloskee Bay; mosquitoes on Sandfly Island trail, especially in the summer

Gulf Coast VC: N25° 50.730' W81° 23.234'

Sandfly Island: N25° 49.395' W81° 23.987'

Start turn for loop: N25° 48.957' W81° 23.959'

Hairpin at bottom of loop: N25° 48.859' W81° 23.898'

Oyster beds at Chokoloskee Bay: N25° 49.510' W81° 23.412'

Maps & Charts: USGS Quadrangle *Everglades City, FL* 7.5-minute; NOAA Nautical Chart 11430; Waterproof Chart 41; a trip map may be available from Gulf Coast VC, or download one from **nps.gov/ever/planyourvisit.**

▶ **Description** While an out-and-back to explore Sandfly Island is a great trip, paddling the loop provides an opportunity to return on a quiet side channel through mangrove islands and around the oyster beds that line the south rim of Chokoloskee Bay.

The loop you make is not around Sandfly Island itself, but around the large mangrove island across the pass from the Sandfly dock.

As with all paddles in the proximity of the Gulf, consider tides when you plan this trip. A falling tide will ease your paddle to Sandfly Island. A rising tide will help you paddle home. In either case, paddling against the tide will take more time and effort. If you make your return trip into Chokoloskee Bay at low tide, you may find the oyster beds impassable and have to go back the way you came.

▶ **Route** When guests stop at the Gulf Coast VC asking for information about places to paddle, one of the maps they receive is the Sandfly Island Loop route. Rangers have told us that paddlers frequently get confused on this trip because when they leave Sandfly Island heading south, they miss the turn for the loop back. This description should clear up some of the uncertainty.

From your put-in at the Gulf Coast VC, paddle 1.5 miles south across Chokoloskee Bay to USCG marker 2 (red) and

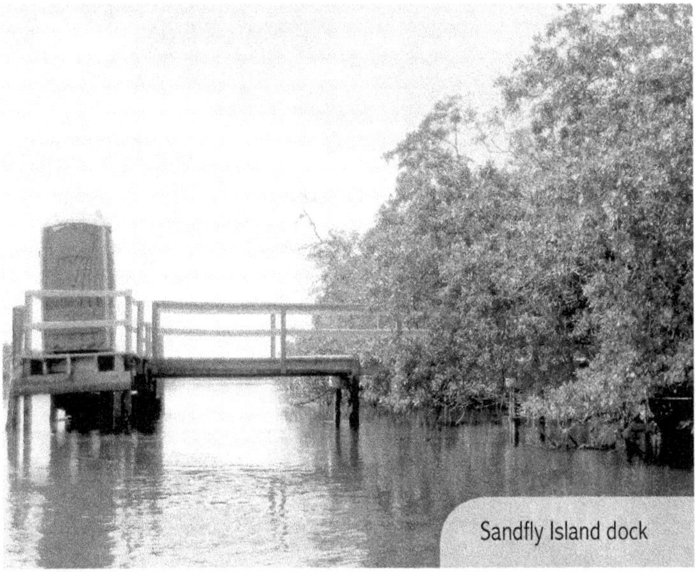

Sandfly Island dock

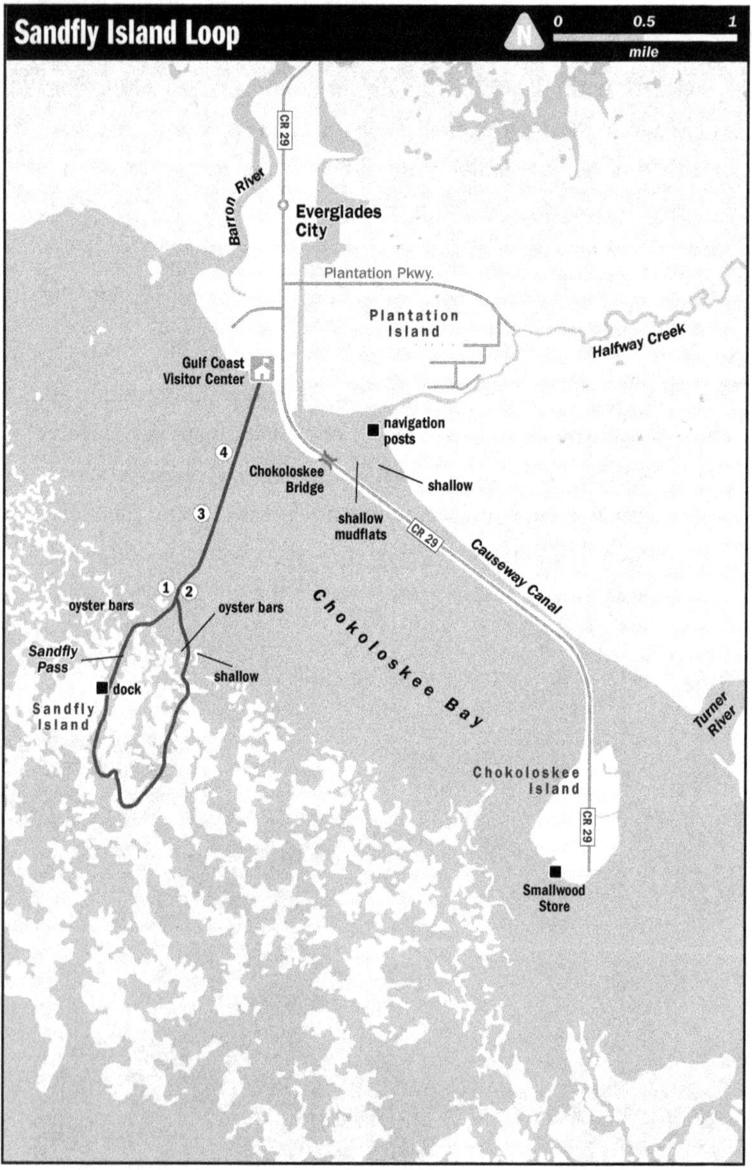
Sandfly Island Loop
N
0
0.5
1
mile
CR 29
Barron River
Everglades City
Plantation Pkwy.
Plantation Island
Halfway Creek
Gulf Coast Visitor Center
navigation posts
4
Chokoloskee Bridge
shallow
3
shallow mudflats
CR 29
Causeway Canal
1
2
oyster bars
oyster bars
Chokoloskee Bay
Sandfly Pass
shallow
dock
Sandfly Island
Turner River
Chokoloskee Island
CR 29
Smallwood Store

enter Sandfly Pass. Because of shallow water, marker 2 and other Coast Guard markers lead you into the pass a bit to the left (east) of where you see the dock and privy. Continue down the pass, pull up to the shore next to the Sandfly dock, and tie your boat securely to a mangrove. The dock itself can be quite slippery, and the water in the pass moves fast.

Explore Sandfly, created 2,000 years ago by the Calusa, who deposited millions of clam and oyster shells to form a horseshoe-shaped island. This shell mound has had a more recent history as well, as early Everglades pioneers lived and farmed on the island. Take the 1-mile nature trail to see remnants of pioneer activity and particularly to explore the vegetation on this hardwood hammock. (See the previous Sandfly Island route description, on page 129, for more detailed information about this unique island.)

When you leave Sandfly Island, continue 0.5 mile south down the pass and watch for the turn to the left (east) that is the start of the turn for your trip back. If you turn too soon, you will shortly come to a dead end. Just come out and continue on to the next left turn. A landmark that may help you locate the turn is the scrap of shell beach that you will see on the right (west) side of Sandfly Pass shortly before you turn. If you travel down the pass so far that the channel opens up wide, you have gone too far. Turn back.

Another way to be sure you're turning at the right place is to keep an eye on what is behind you. When the Sandfly dock disappears behind you, you are already entering your hairpin turn. Keep to the left of the pass, paddling east along the shore of the island that you will be circling, and then turn sharply to the north.

Assuming that you have gotten yourself onto the loop, you are now on your way back to Chokoloskee Bay. Continue north through this quieter pass, paddling among small islands and taking care to weave around the oyster beds as you reenter the bay.

Travel north across the bay to the ranger station and to your takeout at the Gulf Coast VC, where you began this loop.

SMALLWOOD STORE LOOP

SMALLWOOD STORE LOOP

Distance: 7-mile loop

Paddle Time: 2.5–3 hours, plus time to visit the store/museum

Hazards: Muddy launch at low tide; strong tidal flow under Chokoloskee Bridge; heavy seasonal powerboat traffic; potential wind, waves, and oyster beds in Chokoloskee Bay

Gulf Coast VC: N25° 50.730' W81° 23.234'

South end of Chokoloskee Island: N25° 48.537' W81° 21.442'

Historic Smallwood Store: N25° 48.576' W81° 21.743'

Maps & Charts: USGS Quadrangles *Everglades City, FL* 7.5-minute, *Chokoloskee, FL* 7.5-minute; NOAA Nautical Chart 11430; Waterproof Chart 41

▶ **Description** Kayaking or canoeing this loop is an excellent way to do some bird-watching in the Chokoloskee Causeway Canal, explore the Historic Smallwood Store on Chokoloskee Island, and experience the wildlife in Chokoloskee Bay. It's a great short paddle for those who want to stay close to civilization.

The Chokoloskee Causeway was built in 1955 to connect the community on Chokoloskee Island with the mainland at Everglades City. Excavated when material was dredged up to build the causeway, the canal now allows boaters to get to the Turner and Lopez rivers without having to contend with the oyster beds and shallow water in Chokoloskee Bay. Lined with mangroves on the east and mudbanks on the west at low tide, the canal can be a bird-watcher's paradise when the mudbanks are exposed. Snowy egrets, night herons, and little blue and great blue herons poke in the shallows for small fish and mollusks, while little green herons fish from the low branches of mangroves.

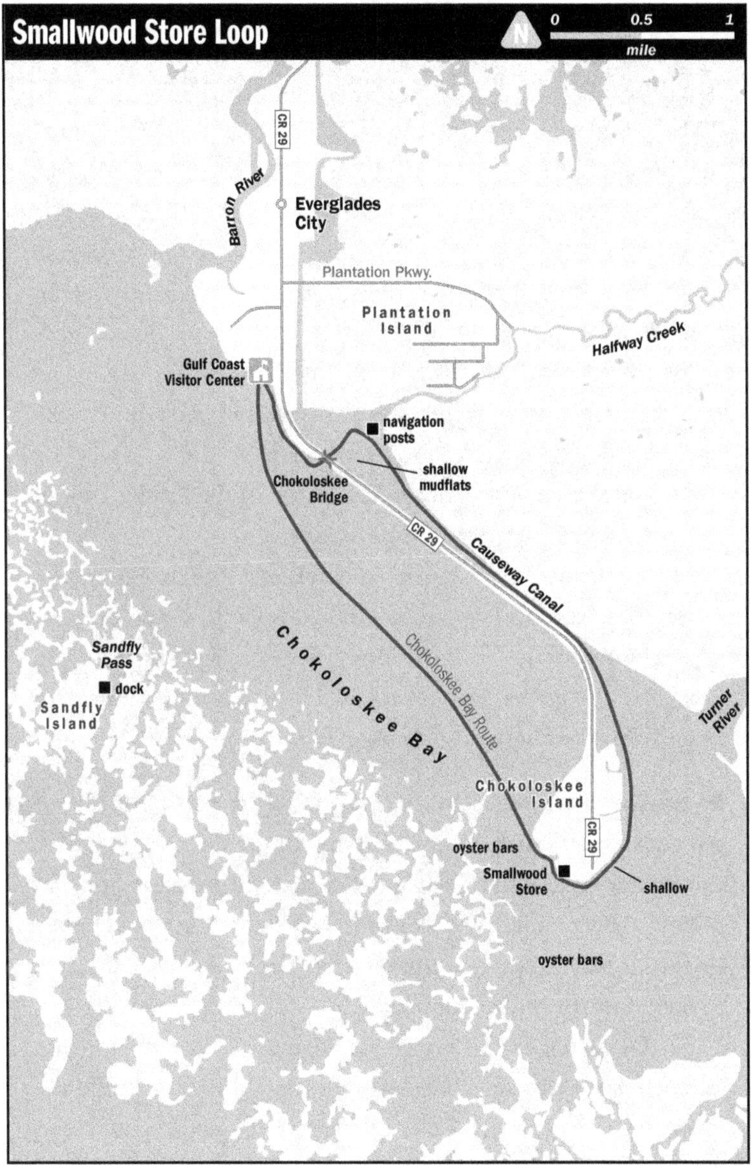
Smallwood Store Loop
N
0
0.5
1
mile
CR 29
Barron River
Everglades City
Plantation Pkwy.
Plantation Island
Halfway Creek
Gulf Coast Visitor Center
navigation posts
shallow mudflats
Chokoloskee Bridge
CR 29
Causeway Canal
Chokoloskee Bay
Chokoloskee Bay Route
Sandfly Pass
dock
Sandfly Island
Turner River
Chokoloskee Island
CR 29
oyster bars
Smallwood Store
shallow
oyster bars

Dry land is scarce in the Everglades. But more than 2,000 years ago, the Calusa mound builders constructed Chokoloskee Island (see page 248), a large shell mound reaching a height of 20 feet. Centuries after the era of the Calusa, early settlers found high ground for settlement on this mound. John Weeks was the first white man to settle Chokoloskee, in 1870. Within the next 25 years other families arrived, setting up homes and farms, and in 1891 the Everglades's first postmaster, C. G. McKinney, served here. A school was established in 1898, and Ted Smallwood built a store in 1906. Many of the year-round residents of the island today are relatives of these early pioneers, but snowbirds make their winter homes here now, too, lured by the mild climate and first-rate fishing grounds in the waters of the nearby Gulf of Mexico, as well as the interior bays and rivers.

Listed in the National Register of Historic Places, the Smallwood Store is now a museum and is worth a stop on your trip, affording you the opportunity to get a feel for what life was like in an earlier time on Chokoloskee Island. For more on Historic Smallwood Store, see page 260.

▶ **Route** To begin your loop, launch from the north side of the Gulf Coast VC in Everglades City. In the dry season (winter and spring), try not to launch at low tide, as the mud can be thigh deep. Paddle 0.5 mile south along the shoreline to the Chokoloskee Bridge, turning left (east) to pass under it. The tidal flow is especially strong under the bridge, so paddling is easiest on a rising tide.

Once under the bridge, turn right (southeast) into the Chokoloskee Causeway Canal. If the tide is low, stay to the left (east) side of the channel. Paddle 2 miles down the canal, watching for powerboats, until the channel opens into Chokoloskee Bay. Chokoloskee Island lies to the south. Cross to the island and follow the shoreline south to circle it. You will pass homes, marinas, RV communities, and tiki huts. About 1 mile around, you will come to the Historic Smallwood Store, with a small sand-and-shell beach to the south side. Pull up on the beach, being sure to tie up to a tree so your boat doesn't float away on the tide, and for a small fee, pay a visit to this fascinating museum. Much has been left just as it was when the store was still operational, with documents, photographs, and small displays added for historical depth. You can view the continuously running video clips of early resident and memoir writer Totch Brown talking about the way things used to be. The shop here sells soft drinks, books, and souvenirs.

When you leave Historic Smallwood Store, continue north around the island and head northwest across Chokoloskee Bay to the visitor center, keeping an eye out for oyster beds. Watch for the dolphins, manatees, mullet, and ospreys that make these waters their home.

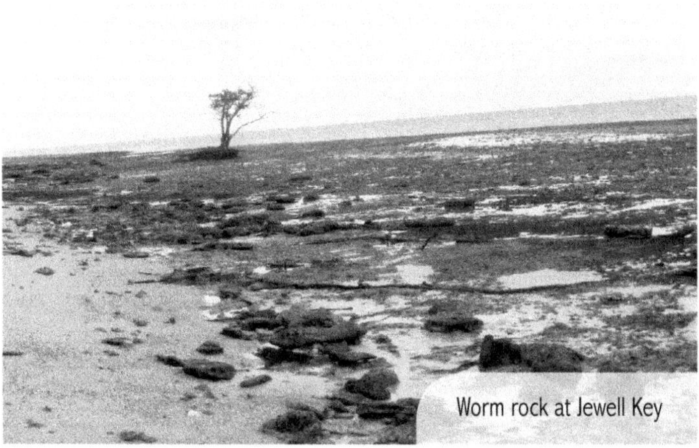

Worm rock at Jewell Key

OVERNIGHT PADDLES—EVERGLADES CITY AREA

HURDDLES CREEK LOOP

HURDDLES CREEK LOOP

Distance: 8.5 miles one-way to Crooked Creek Chickee, plus 8 miles return via Lopez River

Paddle Time: 3.5 hours one-way to Crooked Creek Chickee, plus 3.5 hours return via Lopez River

Hazards: Muddy launch at low tide; strong tidal flow under the Chokoloskee Bridge; heavy seasonal powerboat traffic and potential wind, waves, and oyster beds in Chokoloskee Bay

Gulf Coast VC: N25° 50.730' W81° 23.234'

Turner River: N25° 49.204' W81° 21.015'

WW marker 125: N25° 48.123' W81° 17.589'

Crooked Creek Chickee: N25° 47.785' W81° 17.922'

WW marker 126: N25° 47.686' W81° 17.816'

Lopez River Campsite: N25° 47.275' W81° 18.374'

WW marker 127: N25° 47.320' W81° 20.201'

Chokoloskee Island: N25° 48.537' W81° 21.442'

Maps & Charts: USGS Quadrangle *Chokoloskee, FL* 7.5-minute*; NOAA Nautical Chart 11430; Waterproof Chart 41 (*The short beginning and ending sections included in *Everglades City, FL* 7.5-minute are not necessary if this guidebook is followed.)

▶ **Description** This is an overnight loop from Everglades City through a series of inland rivers and bays to Crooked Creek Chickee, with a return trip down the Lopez River and across Chokoloskee Bay. The journey takes you away from the Gulf and into the interior of the park through quiet rivers, bays, and creeks. You will spend the night on a chickee and return down the Lopez River, stopping to explore the historic Lopez homesite. (Whether you stay at the Crooked Creek Chickee or at the Lopez River Campsite, be sure to make the mandatory

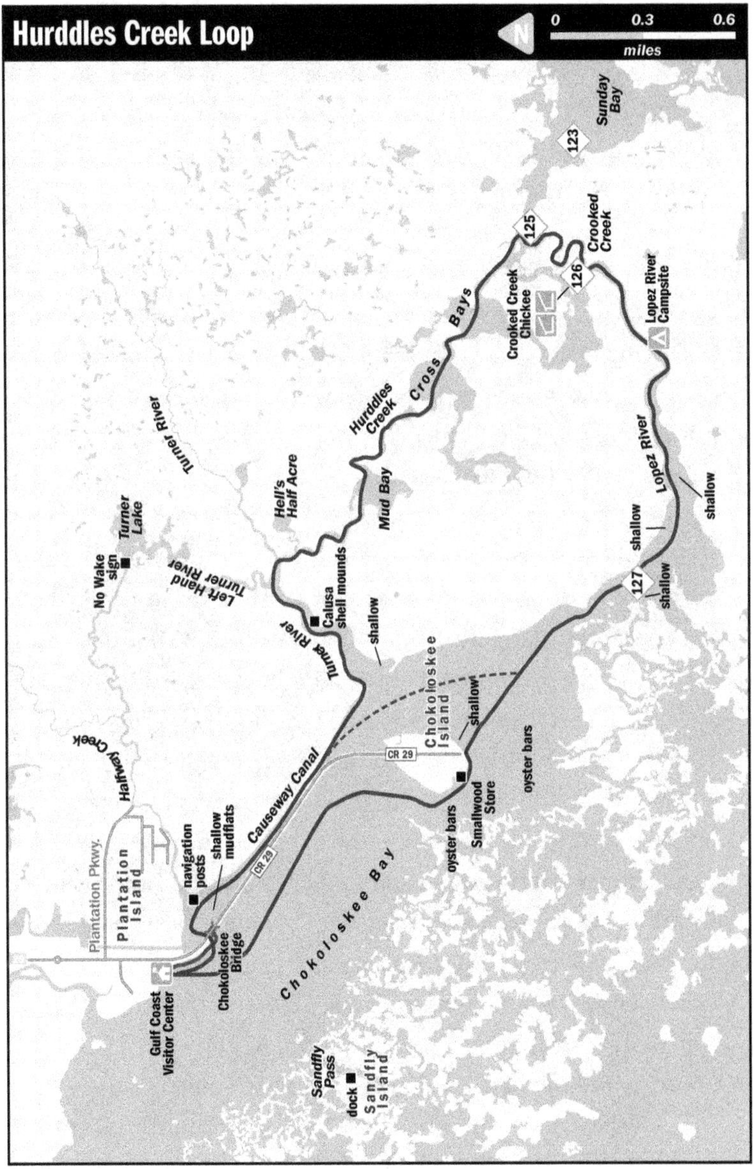
Hurddles Creek Loop
N
0
0.3
0.6
miles
Sunday Bay
123
125
Crooked Creek
126
Crooked Creek Chickee
Lopez River Campsite
Lopez River
shallow
shallow
127
shallow
Bays
Cross
Hurddles Creek
Mud Bay
Hell's Half Acre
Turner River
Turner Lake
No Wake sign
Left Hand Turner River
Calusa shell mounds
shallow
Turner River
Chokoloskee Island
shallow
CR 29
Smallwood Store
oyster bars
oyster bars
Causeway Canal
Halfway Creek
Plantation Pkwy.
Plantation Island
navigation posts
shallow mudflats
CR 29
Chokoloskee Bay
Chokoloskee Bridge
Gulf Coast Visitor Center
Sandfly Pass
dock
Sandfly Island

backcountry camping reservations in person at the visitor center within 24 hours before you launch.)

▶ **Route** Launch from the ramp at the Gulf Coast VC in Everglades City and head south 0.5 mile along the shoreline to the Chokoloskee Bridge. It is preferable to launch on a rising tide that will carry you under the bridge rather than fighting an outgoing tide. Paddle east under the bridge and turn right (south) into the Causeway Canal. If you paddle at low tide, stay to the left (east) bank, where there is a deeper channel, but watch for powerboats. As you paddle this channel, dredged when the causeway was constructed, you will see a variety of wading birds and hear the call of ospreys as they fish these waters.

At the end of the channel, Chokoloskee Bay opens before you, with Chokoloskee Island to the southwest. Continue traveling southeast along the shoreline to the entrance to Turner River. Turn left (northeast) into Turner River (see page 263), named for Captain Richard Bushrod Turner, who homesteaded on one of the Calusa shell mounds on the banks of this river. The mounds lie on the right bank, about 0.25 mile inside the river's mouth.

Paddle northeast up the river, curving east, then north, and then east. At 1.5 miles from the mouth of the river, the Left Hand Turner River branches off to the left (north). But you stay on the main Turner River, traveling east for 0.25 mile, where the Turner becomes much smaller and branches off to the left (northeast). Do not take the small side streams to the left that head into Hell's Half Acre. Instead, stay right, on the wider Hurddles Creek, remaining in the main channel for 1.25 miles.

When the creek opens into Mud Bay, immediately turn northeast (left), leaving the body of Mud Bay to your right. (Do not paddle northwest into a dead-end stream.) Continue northeast in Hurddles Creek, which soon makes a sharp bend south and then runs east for 1 mile until it enters the first of the two Cross Bays. Paddle across this bay traveling east, and once again enter Hurddles Creek. At 0.25 mile farther, Hurddles Creek enters the second Cross Bay. Again, paddle east across the bay, and enter the last stretch of Hurddles Creek, where it continues for 1 mile to marker 125, which indicates the entrance to Crooked Creek. Turn right (south) into the creek and travel for 1.25 miles until you see the Lopez River in front of you. Crooked Creek Chickee is behind a mangrove island on your right. To return the next day, rejoin Crooked Creek where it meets the Lopez River at marker 126. Head southwest down the river for 1 mile. You will see the Lopez River Campsite on the left (south) side of the river. Consider stopping at this historic site to explore the cistern and other remains of the homesite of Spanish pioneer Gregorio Lopez. In the late 1800s, Lopez settled here to fish, hunt, trap, and raise a family; some of his relatives still live on Chokoloskee.

Also, if you were not able to reserve Crooked Creek Chickee for your overnight stay, Lopez River Campsite is a good alternative (see the description on page 230).

Paddling on to your takeout, continue down the Lopez River, watching for powerboat traffic. At the mouth of the river, turn northwest (right) to marker 127. Head into the bay toward Chokoloskee Island. If the tide is low and the oyster beds and mudbanks are visible, pass to the right (east) side of Chokoloskee Island and return to the visitor center via the canal that parallels the causeway. If there is sufficient water in the bay, and particularly if the tide is coming in, since it is hard to paddle against the tide under the Chokoloskee Bridge, finish the loop by paddling along the west side of Chokoloskee Island. Pass the Historic Smallwood Store (see page 260), and head northwest to the Gulf Coast VC. Watch for leaping mullet, as well as the manatees and dolphins that enjoy Chokoloskee Bay.

INDIAN KEY PASS

INDIAN KEY PASS

Distance: 7.5 miles one-way from Everglades City to Picnic Key; 8.5 miles one-way from Everglades City to Tiger Key; 10.5 miles one-way from Everglades City to Camp LuLu Key; thus 15–21 miles round-trip

Paddle Time: 3–7 hours, depending on tides

Hazards: Muddy launch at low tide; heavy seasonal powerboat traffic; strong tidal flow to and from the Gulf; worm rock on keys at low tide; heavy morning and evening mosquitoes on the keys when camping in the summer

Gulf Coast VC: N25° 50.730' W81° 23.234'

USCG marker 24: N25° 50.394' W81° 24.448'

USCG beacon 7: N25° 49.698' W81° 26.401'

Indian Key: N25° 49.559' W81° 29.126'

Picnic Key: N25° 49.386' W81° 29.052'

Tiger Key: N25° 49.716' W81° 29.501'

Camp Lulu Key: N25° 50.113' W81° 30.409'

Maps & Charts: USGS Quadrangle *Everglades City, FL* 7.5-minute; NOAA Nautical Chart 11430; Waterproof Chart 41

▶ **Description** Indian Key Pass is a direct, well-marked passage from Everglades City to the Gulf of Mexico, cutting through mangrove islands, shell mounds, and spoil banks deposited as the channel was dredged. This paddle offers you the opportunity to explore the mangrove habitat and the variety of life that inhabits these waters from the bay to the Gulf. You will also have the experience of camping on the beach on the Gulf of Mexico on Picnic, Tiger, or Camp Lulu Key. (Just remember that reservations must be made in person at the Gulf Coast VC within 24 hours of launch for all backcountry camping. However, as Camp Lulu Key is outside the park's boundaries, you do not need a reservation to camp there.)

Tides are especially important to your safety and enjoyment when you make this trip. Paddling the Indian Key Pass

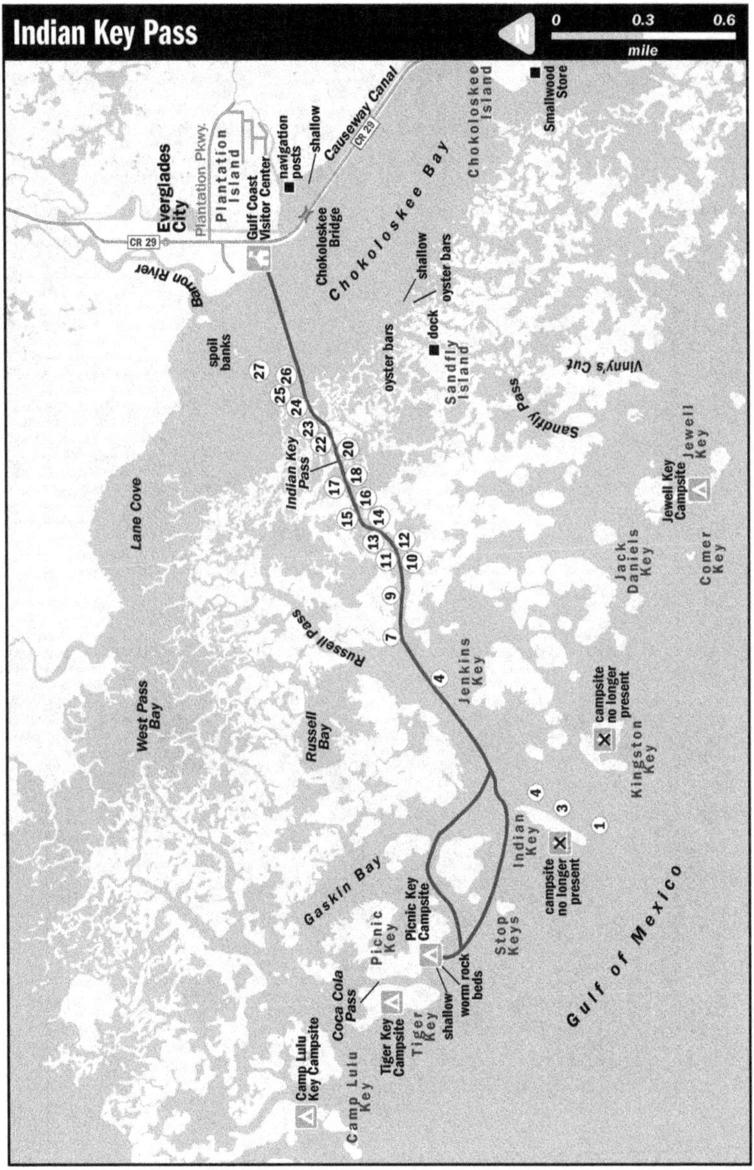
Indian Key Pass
N
0
0.3
0.6
mile
Everglades City
Plantation Pkwy.
Plantation Island
CR 29
Gulf Coast Visitor Center
navigation posts
shallow
Causeway Canal
Chokoloskee Bridge
Chokoloskee Bay
Chokoloskee Island
Smallwood Store
Barron River
spoil banks
oyster bars
shallow
oyster bars
dock
Sandfly Island
Vinny's Cut
Sandfly Pass
Jewell Key
Jewell Key Campsite
Indian Key Pass
Lane Cove
Russell Pass
Jack Daniels Key
Comer Key
Jenkins Key
West Pass Bay
Russell Bay
campsite no longer present
Kingston Key
Indian Key
campsite no longer present
Gaskin Bay
Picnic Key
Picnic Key Campsite
Stop Keys
Gulf of Mexico
Coca Cola Pass
Tiger Key Campsite
Tiger Key
shallow
worm rock beds
Camp Lulu Key Campsite
Camp Lulu Key

route can be quick and easy, or if the tide is against you, it can be strenuous and take twice as long. It all depends on the tides and the wind. Prior to launch, be sure to get tide charts from the visitor center or download them from **saltwatertides.com.**

Generally, as noted in "Mind the Tides," on page 7, one moderate low tide is followed by a high tide and then a more extreme low tide. The best time to launch from Everglades City is at full high tide, when the water starts flowing back into the Gulf. Go with the flow, as they say.

On the other hand, if you start your paddle at low tide, you will be battling the water that is coming back to Everglades City from the Gulf of Mexico, and your trip can take 6 hours down the pass rather than 3. If the wind is coming from the southwest up the channel, the paddle out will be even more difficult.

Also, if you paddle in the winter and spring dry seasons, when there is not as much water in the Glades as in summer and fall, you might be walking out into thigh-deep mud to load and

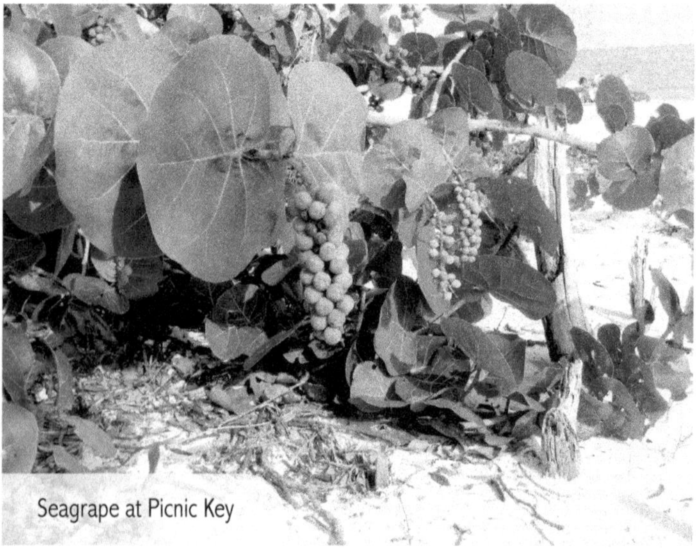

Seagrape at Picnic Key

launch your boat from Everglades City. (For alternative launch sites at Chokoloskee Island, see Appendix 2, Launch Sites, on page 269, and Appendix 4, Resource Overview, on page 278.)

Ideally, you should make your return trip on the incoming tide, when the water comes back to Everglades City from the Gulf.

For all the challenge that tides can bring to your travels, they also can bring delight. The lowest low tides on Picnic Key lay bare large expanses of worm rock (see page 264) and tidepools that are great places to discover the tiny crabs, mollusks, and other sea life that are exposed during this brief period in the cycle of the sea. Note that the tides at Picnic and Tiger keys are 1.5–2 hours different from those at Everglades City, with high tides arriving at the keys earlier and low tides arriving later.

▶ **Route** From the launch at the Gulf Coast VC at Everglades City, you will be able to spot the red and green markers that indicate the entrance to the channel for Indian Key Pass. (As you launch, don't get confused by the markers on the right—north—that guide boats into the Barron River.) You may also note a tour boat traveling in or out of the Indian Key channel, and that will give you a visual indicator of the location of the pass.

As the most direct route from the marinas of the Barron River to the Gulf, Indian Key Pass is heavily used by fishing boats and park service tour boats, so use caution and stay well to the side of the marked channel.

Once launched, travel west across Chokoloskee Bay, passing USCG marker 27 to your right, followed by marker 26, and then marker 24 located next to a spoil bank with the sign EVERGLADES NATIONAL PARK BOUNDARY, SPECIAL REGULATIONS APPLY. Travel from marker 23 to marker 9 through the pass, jogging south and west.

The bends in the channel are marked by beacons. At beacon 7 you will veer southwest where the pass widens toward the Gulf. Pass marker 6 and continue in a southwesterly direction toward Indian Key, keeping the large mangrove island to your right (north). Indian Key lies directly ahead of you with markers 3 and 4 visible on the key's south side.

If the winds and tides are in your favor and the waves are not too strong, you might choose to continue down the pass toward Indian Key en route to Picnic Key: turn slightly right (northwest) as you approach Indian Key and keep paddling northwest as you pass around or between the Stop Keys to reach Picnic Key.

If the waves are heavy, however, back between marker 6 and Indian Key, you can turn harder right (north) into Gaskin Bay. The large mangrove island will be to your right with a smaller mangrove island to your left. Pass between these two mangrove islands and then curve west into the unnamed channel leading out to the Gulf. Picnic Key lies to your right when approached from this direction. Also, traveling through this bit of Gaskin Bay can be a treat because dolphins (see page 250) seem to like this spot and can often be seen fishing and splashing where the Gulf enters the bay.

The campsite on Picnic Key occupies a sandy beach on the southwest side of the island. Note the Picnic Key sign and a privy on the western end of the beach. Additional camping is located around the western end of the island.

If you camp on Tiger Key, just west of Picnic Key, you can choose to pitch your tent on either the western or northern shores. As mentioned above, you also may camp on Camp LuLu Key (northwest of Tiger Key), where no reservations are required. Be aware that, although a campsite is marked on Indian Key on both the NOAA and Waterproof charts, the park service has closed this campsite. You may also read about a campsite at Kingston Key, but that chickee was destroyed by Hurricane Wilma and will not be replaced.

On your return trip after a night on the Gulf, head back toward Indian Key. You can travel east through Gaskin Bay to avoid waves on the Gulf or you can paddle directly southeast along the Gulf. At Indian Key head northeast into Indian Key Pass. Watch for marker 6 and take care at this point to locate beacon 7 for the easterly jog into Indian Key Pass channel. This is the only tricky navigational spot on the route. Be alert so as not to take the left (north) unmarked channel, leading into Russell Pass. Follow the markers back along Indian Key Pass to Chokoloskee Bay, and cross it as you did on your outbound route. Take out at Gulf Coast VC.

JEWELL KEY

JEWELL KEY

Distance: 4.5 miles one-way

Paddle Time: 3–4 hours each way, depending on tides

Hazards: Muddy launch at low tide; heavy seasonal powerboat traffic; strong tidal flow in Sandfly Pass; potential wind and waves in Chokoloskee Bay and the Gulf; heavy mosquitoes in the summer when camping on Jewell Key

Gulf Coast VC: N25° 50.730' W81° 23.234'

Sandfly Island: N25° 49.395' W81° 23.987'

Mouth of Sandfly Pass at the Gulf: N25° 48.027' W81° 24.695'

Jewell Key: N25° 47.312' W81° 25.113'

Maps & Charts: USGS Quadrangle *Everglades City, FL* 7.5-minute; NOAA Nautical Chart 11430; Waterproof Chart 41

▶ **Description** With careful planning, this might also be a 9-mile day trip, but be sure to return on a rising tide if you do not intend to stay overnight.

The route takes you down Sandfly Pass from Chokoloskee Bay to the Gulf of Mexico. Along the way you pass historic

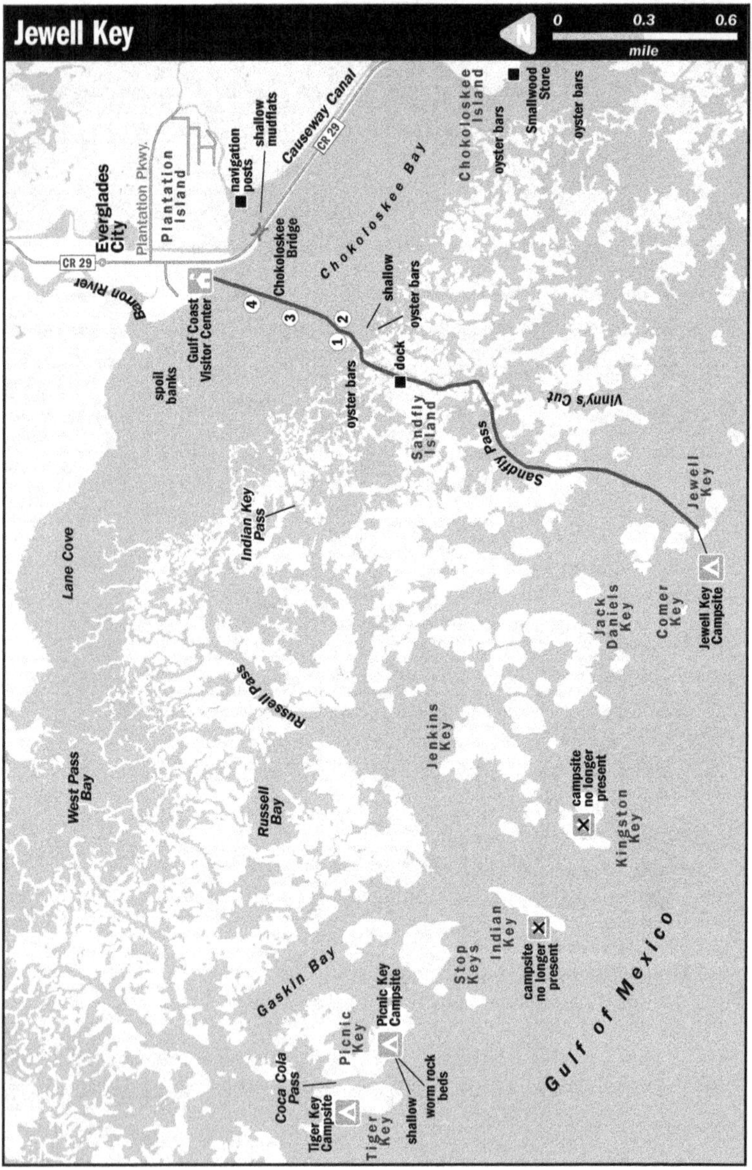
Jewell Key
0
0.3
0.6
mile
Everglades City
CR 29
Plantation Pkwy.
Plantation Island
navigation posts
shallow mudflats
Causeway Canal
CR 29
Chokoloskee Bridge
Chokoloskee Bay
Chokoloskee Island
Smallwood Store
oyster bars
oyster bars
oyster bars
Barron River
Gulf Coast Visitor Center
spoil banks
4
3
2
1
shallow
oyster bars
oyster bars
dock
Sandfly Island
Vinny's Cut
Sandfly Pass
Jewell Key
Jewell Key Campsite
Indian Key Pass
Lane Cove
Jack Daniels Key
Comer Key
Russell Pass
Jenkins Key
West Pass Bay
Russell Bay
campsite no longer present
Kingston Key
Indian Key
campsite no longer present
Stop Keys
Gaskin Bay
Picnic Key
Picnic Key Campsite
Coca Cola Pass
Tiger Key Campsite
Tiger Key
shallow
worm rock beds
Gulf of Mexico

Sandfly Island, where you can stop and explore the 1-mile nature trail, but watch the tides. You will want to paddle the pass out to the Gulf on a falling tide or you will be fighting the current all the way. (For more on Sandfly Island, see the Sandfly Island and Sandfly Island Loop day trips, pages 129 and 132, respectively.)

Your destination is the beach campsite at Jewell Key. Set up your tent at the designated camping area on the north end of the island (*not* on the Gulf side) and explore the tidepools at low tide or relax on the beach. For every Everglades paddle you should carry binoculars, but for this one especially; don't forget to pack them as this route offers excellent birding opportunities.

Jewell Key is separated from its neighboring key by a narrow channel where herons and egrets fish from the mangrove roots hanging over the water. Brown pelicans dive in the cove at the south end of the camping beach. And Comer Key, northwest of Jewell Key, is a scrap of sand that, depending on the tide and the season, is visited by white pelicans and a variety of shorebirds. It is odd to think that at one time Comer Key had trees and other vegetation and was the location of the dock and fishing camp of former Alabama Governor Braxton Bragg Comer. In 1960 Hurricane Donna swept it all away.

Although the beach at Jewell Key is small, beachcombing is excellent at low tide, with an expanse of sand where shells and worm rock are exposed. A walk around the north side of the island from the camping area gives more opportunities for exploration and views of twisted buttonwoods. Be sure to wear shoes, for the worm rock is hard and the oyster shells sharp.

▶ **Route** Launch from the Gulf Coast VC at high tide, when the outgoing current can carry you along to the Gulf. Travel 1.5 miles south across Chokoloskee Bay. You should be able to see the dock and privy on Sandfly Island. Do not confuse Sandfly Pass

Gulf landing

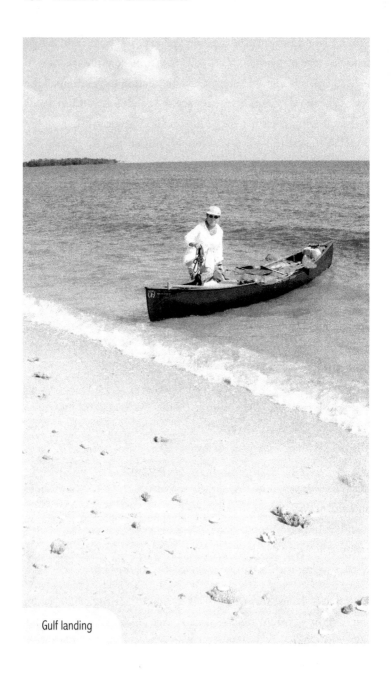

with Indian Key Pass to the right (northwest), where the park service tour boats go.

At USCG marker 2 (red) you will enter Sandfly Pass, and the Sandfly Island dock will be 0.5 mile down on your right. The trick to navigating this whole route to the Gulf is to follow the main channel with the strongest current. You will pass bays to the left and right and an alternate pass to the southeast, but stay in the main channel.

From the Sandfly Island dock, you will paddle approximately 0.5 mile south until the pass bends to the right (southwest). We think of this as "the elbow" on the charts. Paddle southwest for 1 mile until the pass again turns south. At this point you will see the Gulf of Mexico before you.

When you leave Sandfly Pass and head into the Gulf, Jewell Key lies 1 mile ahead of you out in the Gulf. What looks like one large island at a distance is really a cluster of islands. As you paddle closer you will pass two islands on your right (west), one very small and the next larger. At this point you should see the beach and privy at Jewell Key. The next island on your right (west) is Jewell Key's sister island. Pass that island, and land on the beach at Jewell Key. Be aware that the beach drops off sharply here.

The next day, take a rising tide to return to Everglades City. Paddle northeast to Sandfly Pass, then north for 0.5 mile, then northeast for 1 mile, and, turning north at "the elbow," paddle the remaining mile back to Chokoloskee Bay. Head north across the bay to your takeout at the visitor center.

Dock at Bear Lake Canoe Trail

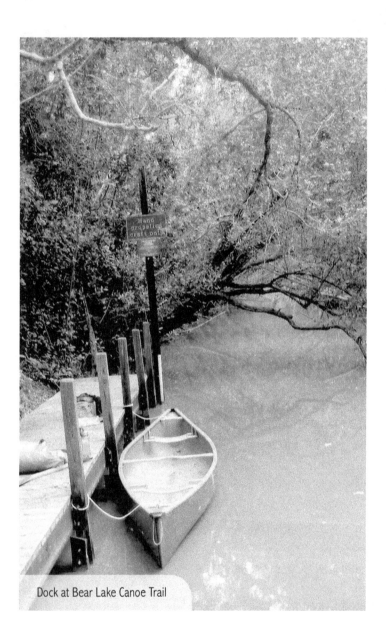

Part Three:

South Everglades Day & Overnight Paddles

Just as in the North Everglades, the South Everglades offers many opportunities for paddlers to experience waterways, flora, fauna, campsites, and chickees—even if all you have is a few hours or time for an overnight escape.

The nine excursions described in this section guide you through twisty mangrove tunnels, wet prairies, wildlife-rich lakes and ponds, and beautiful Florida Bay. You will have diverse choices—from an easy trip down the Buttonwood Canal to testing your paddling skills as you weave your way through serpentine channels that lead to Noble Hammock. You will be following old airboat trails, making your way to the site of an old Prohibition-era whiskey still, or exploring the hidden passages used by gator hunters and by 19th- and early 20th-century plumers harvesting bird feathers primarily for ladies' hats. Whichever trail you choose, you will be traveling through unique ecosystems and sites of Florida history.

All of the paddles in this section originate from the Flamingo area, near the south entrance to Everglades National Park. Conveniently located, this entrance lies just 11 miles west of the town of Homestead.

Like the adventures included in the North Everglades day trips and overnights (beginning on page 118), each paddle here is a loop or an out-and-back: no shuttles are required. Canoe and kayak rentals are available from the concessionaire in Flamingo and from local outfitters. (See Appendix 2, Launch Sites, on page 269; Appendix 3, Outfitters, Suppliers, & Canoe/Kayak Rentals, on page 275; and Appendix 4, Resource Overview, on page 278.)

PLAN AHEAD

While the 99-mile Wilderness Waterway expedition described in Part One of this book requires extensive planning, an Everglades day or overnight outing also necessitates careful thought.

The Wilderness Waterway "Trip Preparation" section, on page 32, provides a good framework from which you can modify your supplies for a day trip or an overnight. If you are paddling in the summer months, consult Part Four, Summer Paddling, on page 201, as well.

THE NONNEGOTIABLE BASICS

As we repeat throughout this guidebook, you should not shirk the requirements for water (1 gallon per person per day), and don't forget snacks, insect repellent, sunscreen, lip balm, a hat, and sunglasses. Check weather predictions and tide tables.

RESERVATIONS

If you plan to camp in the backcountry, you must make reservations—at either the Flamingo or the Gulf Coast Visitor Center—in person within 24 hours of your launch.

DIRECTIONS

To access the park from the east (Miami), take either US 1 or the Florida Turnpike (FL 821) south to Homestead. Here, you can pick up any last-minute provisions that you might need. Inside the park, apart from vending machine fare at Royal Palm, the only place to buy food is a small store with basic snacks and sandwiches at the marina and a café near the visitor center in Flamingo, 38 miles inside the park. (The lodge and restaurant in Flamingo were destroyed in

2005 by Hurricanes Katrina and Wilma. As of this writing they are expected to be rebuilt, pending funding.)

From US 1 in Florida City, turn right (west) onto FL 9336, and drive approximately 2 miles. Turn left in front of Robert Is Here, a famous wayside fruit-and-vegetable market. You may want to stop here for a great Key lime shake or some fruit—or just to have the Robert Is Here experience.

Continue on FL 9336, traveling south. In approximately 2 miles, the route makes a right (west) turn and continues for about 5 miles to the park entrance.

To access the park from the west (Naples), take I-75 (Alligator Alley) east through the first tollbooth to Exit 80, FL 29 south. Travel 17 miles south to FL 41 (the Tamiami Trail). Turn left (east) on FL 41, and drive 58 miles to FL 997 (Krome Avenue). Turn right (south) on Krome Avenue, and continue approximately 22 miles into Homestead and then Florida City. Turn right (west) onto FL 9336, and drive 2 miles to Robert Is Here, the fruit stand described above. Turn left (south) in front of Robert Is Here. In approximately 2 miles, FL 9336 makes a right (west) turn and continues for about 5 miles to the park entrance.

Especially if you are a first-time visitor, you may want to stop at Ernest F. Coe Visitor Center for an introduction to Everglades National Park before continuing on the park road to the entrance station. At the station, you will pay a fee plus a small additional amount to launch your canoe or kayak.

The park road extends 38 miles from the entrance station to the Flamingo VC and Flamingo Marina. To paddle the trails described in this section, you will launch from sites off this park road or from Flamingo at the end of the road on Florida Bay.

DAY PADDLES—FLAMINGO AREA

BEAR LAKE CANOE TRAIL

BEAR LAKE CANOE TRAIL

Distance: 4 miles round-trip

Paddle Time: 3 hours round-trip

Hazards: Low water level at Bear Lake end of trail; possibility of heavy mosquitoes in the rainy season

Launch from access road: N25° 10.461' W80° 55.397'

NPS marker 1: N25° 10.467' W80° 55.474'

Roberts Prairie: N25° 10.472' W80° 56.030'

Calusa shell mounds: N25° 10.461' W80° 56.140'

NPS marker 2: N25° 10.479' W80° 56.831'

NPS marker 3: N25° 10.480' W80° 56.880'

Cutoff to Mud Lake: N25° 10.484' W80° 56.846'

Bear Lake: N25° 10.482' W80° 56.969'

Maps & Charts: USGS Quadrangle *Flamingo, FL* 7.5-minute; NOAA Nautical Chart 11433 or 11451; Waterproof Chart 39; National Geographic Everglades TopoMap; "Mud Lake Loop [Canoe] Trail" map available at the Flamingo VC. (*Note:* Even though the charts indicate that the route will take you all the way to Cape Sable, you will not be able to travel past Bear Lake.)

▶ **Description** Even if seas and winds are high on nearby Florida Bay, they have little influence here, and navigation is easy. There are only two hazards to this trip—a chance of heavy mosquitoes as you wend through this mangrove "tunnel" and the possibility of extremely shallow water as you approach Bear Lake. You can prepare for the mosquitoes by bringing insect repellent (and bug suits, if necessary). If the water gets too shallow as you near Bear Lake, turn around and head back.

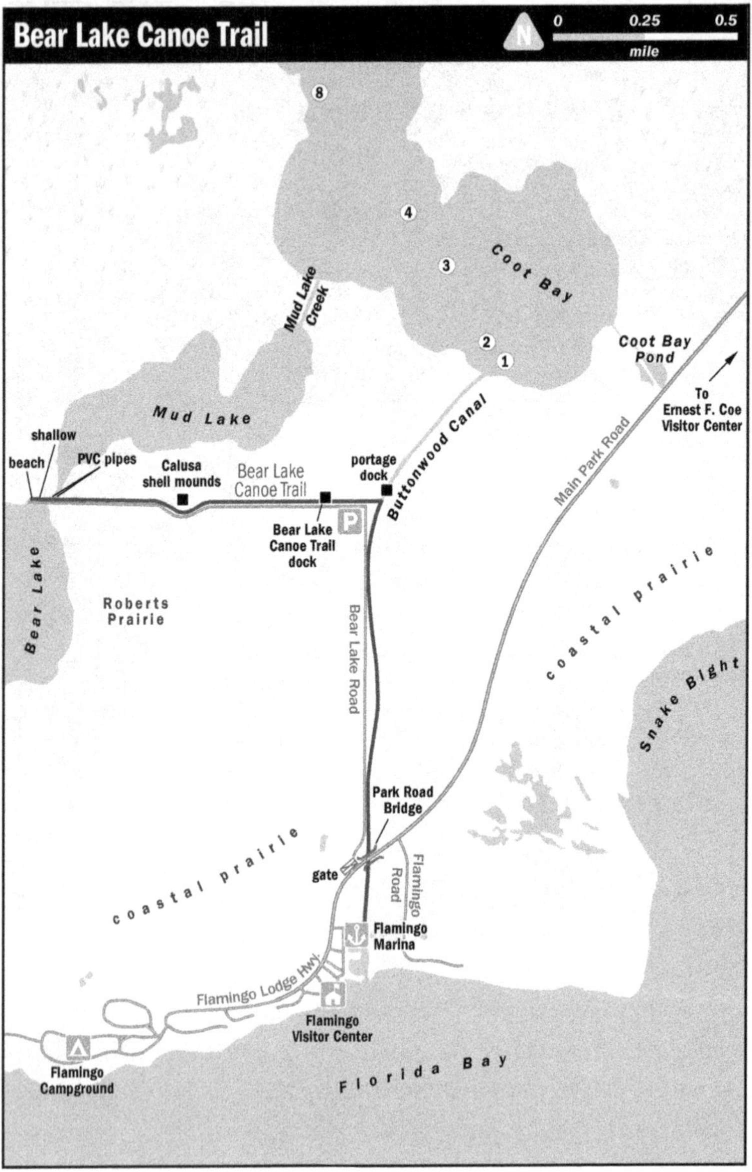
Bear Lake Canoe Trail
0
0.25
0.5
mile
N
8
4
3
2
1
Coot Bay
Coot Bay Pond
Mud Lake Creek
Mud Lake
Buttonwood Canal
To Ernest F. Coe Visitor Center
Main Park Road
shallow
beach
PVC pipes
Calusa shell mounds
Bear Lake Canoe Trail
portage dock
Bear Lake Canoe Trail dock
Bear Lake
Roberts Prairie
Bear Lake Road
coastal prairie
Snake Bight
Park Road Bridge
gate
Flamingo Road
coastal prairie
Flamingo Marina
Flamingo Lodge Hwy.
Flamingo Visitor Center
Flamingo Campground
Florida Bay

Because this route is easy to navigate, you won't need charts here. This is a delightful trip, with a remarkable variety of vegetation en route to your destination: a beautiful spot on a small beach along the shores of Bear Lake. In addition, there is history here, the most recent being when volunteers worked in the summer of 2009, braving heat, fallen trees, and mosquitoes, to reopen the trail after Hurricanes Katrina and Wilma made it impassable. In the 1920s, dredgemen originally dug this channel, known as the Homestead Canal, to open up Cape Sable for development, and 2,000 years ago the Calusa built shell mounds in the area and constructed canals of their own.

Lawrence Will was one of the original 1920s dredgemen, and he wrote in his memoir, *A Dredgeman of Cape Sable,* of his fascination with the Everglades: "It sort of grows on you. It really does! Yet we had our troubles too, insects, sores, boils, balky engines, a boiler explosion, sinkings, frustrations and more insects, we had 'em all. But can you believe it, after being there for blamed near a year, when the job was finished, I'd gladly have stayed a little longer."

As you paddle the Bear Lake Canoe Trail, think about those dredgemen who fought mosquitoes and mangroves and mud to scour this channel, as well as the intrepid current-day volunteers who have worked to open up this trail once again for you. And remember that 2,000 years ago the Calusa lived and traveled in the same place where you are paddling today.

▶ **Route** There are two ways to access the Bear Lake Canoe Trail. The gated Bear Lake Road, which provides access to the launch site, lies just across the Park Road Bridge on the right (west), 0.25 mile before you come to the Flamingo Marina. If the gate to the road is open, drive the 2 miles down this dirt road that parallels the Buttonwood Canal to a small parking area, and turn left to take your boat to the dock at the launch site. Return your car to the parking area.

If the gate is closed, launch from the Flamingo Marina, and paddle 2 miles north along the Buttonwood Canal until you come to the Bear Lake Canoe Trail dock on your left. At the end of the dock, the portage to the Bear Lake Canoe Trail is to the *left*. Carry your boat 250 feet down this wide, clear path to the dock at the beginning of the canoe trail. Launch into the mangrove tunnel, where the air is pungent with the smell of sulfur produced by decaying organic matter. If the scent bothers you, don't worry. It will shortly dissipate as you paddle the canal. A hiking trail parallels the south side of the Bear Lake Canoe Trail on the higher ground formed from deposits as the Homestead Canal was dredged. Describing the hiking trail, a National Park Service (NPS) brochure claims that more than 50 different tree species are on this route. So this is not a trip to paddle in a rush; take time to appreciate the lush vegetation all around you. To the left are hardwood hammock species such as the peeling, red-barked gumbo limbo (see page 251), one of the iconic trees of the Everglades. To the right lies a tangle of red and black mangroves, and overhead, sizable air plants adorn the arching buttonwood branches (see page 246).

About 0.5 mile down the canal, you will enter Roberts Prairie; the vegetation on the right changes into a low, yellow-green meadow of sea purslane, dotted with buttonwoods. So far the canal runs straight east to west, but a little more than a mile from your launch, the channel makes a gentle dip to the south before resuming its westerly course. When the original dredgemen in the 1920s discovered a Calusa shell mound in the path of their canal, they detoured around it.

The mound is a bit hard to spot: watch for the slight southwesterly direction of the channel and the humps of higher ground to your right. Look for the trees that are indicative of higher ground, most noticeably the gumbo limbo standing in a mix of vegetation that includes marlberry, stopper, coral bean, the small-leaved white indigoberry, and the broad-leaved pigeon plum.

Paddling west, you will pass white PVC pipes 2 and 3, marking the channel to the right (north) that leads to Mud Lake. Continue west, and soon the canoe trail opens onto Bear Lake to the south. The shelly beach ahead of you makes a good spot to pull up your boat and have lunch. If time permits, you might paddle out into Bear Lake and do some exploring, or walk a bit back along the hiking trail to stretch your legs.

To return, paddle east back down the canal to your take-out, enjoying the company of patient green and little blue herons, ibis, and egrets.

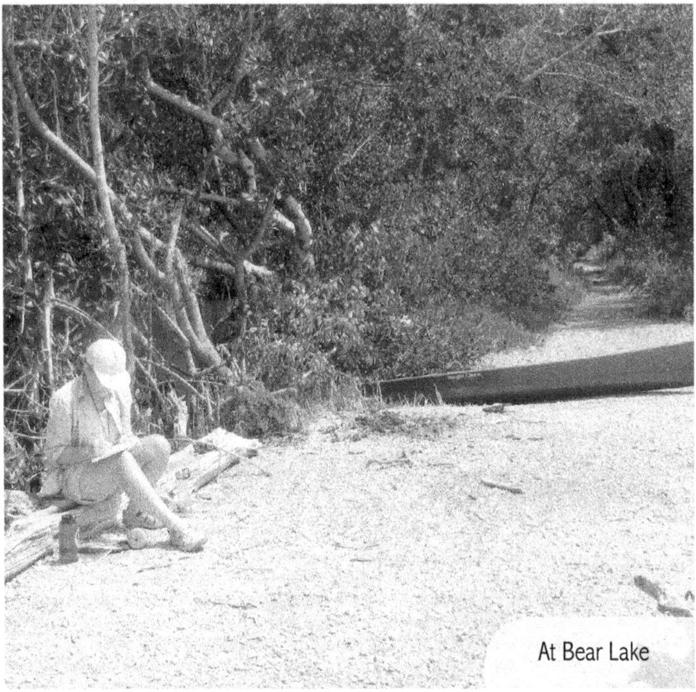

At Bear Lake

MUD LAKE CANOE TRAIL

MUD LAKE CANOE TRAIL

Distance (3 options): 11-mile loop (option 1); 7-mile loop (option 2); 5.5-mile loop, or 9.5-mile loop if launching from Flamingo, (option 3)

Paddle Time: 4–5 hours

Hazards: Powerboats in Coot Bay and the Buttonwood Canal; possible wind on Coot Bay or Mud Lake; mosquitoes in channels, particularly on the Bear Lake Canoe Trail

Flamingo Marina: N25° 8.624' W80° 55.354'

Dock on Buttonwood Canal: N25° 10.474' W80° 55.277'

North end of Buttonwood Canal: N25° 11.012' W80° 54.772'

Entrance to Mud Lake Creek: N25° 11.415' W80° 55.586'

Mud Lake: N25° 11.235' W80° 55.659'

Homestead Canal: N25° 10.627' W80° 56.751'

Bear Lake: N25° 10.486' W80° 56.969'

USCG marker 2: N25° 11.102' W80° 54.726'

Entrance to Coot Bay Pond: N25° 11.085' W80° 53.995'

Launch/takeout on Coot Bay Pond: N25° 10.966' W80° 53.884'

Maps & Charts: USGS Quadrangle *Flamingo, FL 7.5-minute*; NOAA Nautical Chart 11433 (does not show channel between Mud Lake and Bear Lake); Waterproof Chart 39 (does not show channel between Mud Lake and Bear Lake); National Geographic Everglades TopoMap; "Mud Lake Loop [Canoe] Trail" map (option 3) available at the Flamingo VC.

▶ **Description** We present three options for paddling the Mud Lake Canoe Trail, none requiring shuttle service. All three choices will give you the excellent birding experience of Mud Lake and will enable you to travel into sites important in early Flamingo history. The Buttonwood Canal (option 1) and the Bear Lake Canoe Trail (option 3) also give you an opportunity to observe a wide variety of Everglades vegetation.

▶ **The Route: Option 1, via the Buttonwood Canal** This option is a good choice if you plan to rent a canoe or kayak from

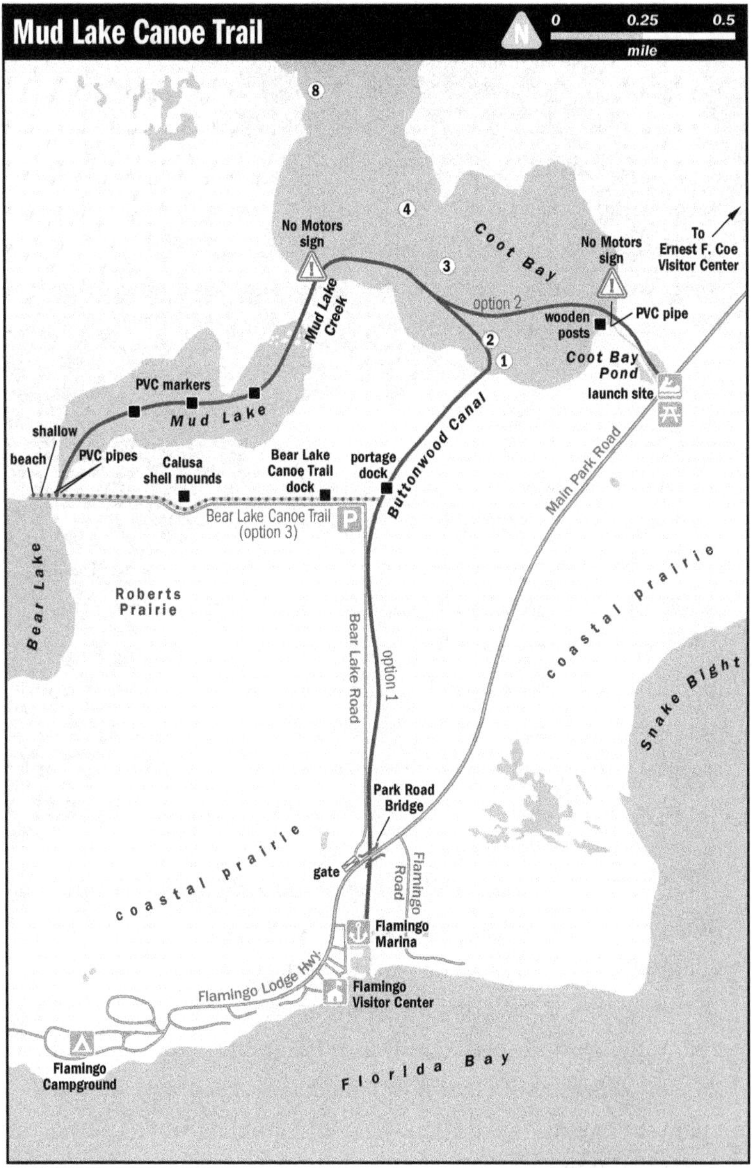
Mud Lake Canoe Trail
0
0.25
0.5
mile
8
4
No Motors sign
Coot Bay
3
No Motors sign
To Ernest F. Coe Visitor Center
option 2
Mud Lake Creek
wooden posts
PVC pipe
2
1
Coot Bay Pond
launch site
PVC markers
Mud Lake
Buttonwood Canal
shallow
beach
PVC pipes
Calusa shell mounds
Bear Lake Canoe Trail dock
portage dock
Main Park Road
Bear Lake Canoe Trail (option 3)
Bear Lake
Roberts Prairie
Bear Lake Road
option 1
coastal prairie
Snake Bight
Park Road Bridge
gate
Flamingo Road
coastal prairie
Flamingo Marina
Flamingo Lodge Hwy.
Flamingo Visitor Center
Flamingo Campground
Florida Bay

the Flamingo Marina. Launch at the Flamingo Marina and paddle 2 miles north on the Buttonwood Canal (see page 246). Watch for American crocodiles and alligators as you travel, and be alert for manatees, which sometimes hang out near the marina.

The manatees can't come up the canal from Florida Bay because the canal has been plugged to stop the ecological damage that would be caused if salt water were allowed to flow into the brackish, fresher water to the north. Instead, these manatees have traveled a long way to the marina from the Gulf of Mexico through the Shark River and Whitewater Bay.

Take time to observe the vegetation that lines the canal. Mangroves stand along the right side of the canal, while the western bank offers a much greater variety of plant life. Look for buttonwoods; purple morning glories; acacia, with its thorns and small yellow flowers; the fat, prickly seedpods of nickerbeans; exotic, invasive Brazilian pepper; air plants in the trees; and the ever-present mangroves. Try to spot the oval leaves and apple-like fruit of the toxic manchineel tree, considered to be the most poisonous tree in the world: *Look but don't touch!* Contact with any part of the plant will cause a yellow, blistering rash, and eating the fruit can be fatal. It is said that one of Columbus's sailors died from eating manchineel "apples."

When you have paddled approximately 1.5 miles up the Buttonwood Canal, you will see ahead of you a dock on the west side of the canal. (The dock marks a portage you will take if you choose option 3, on page 169.) Continue paddling, and at the end of the Buttonwood Canal, turn left (northwest) and follow the near shoreline of Coot Bay. The dolphins you may see feeding in the bay also would have traveled for miles through Whitewater Bay from the Gulf of Mexico. Paddle about 1 mile along the shore to a NO MOTORS sign and the entrance to Mud Lake Creek. The creek is narrow and lined with mangroves, their prop

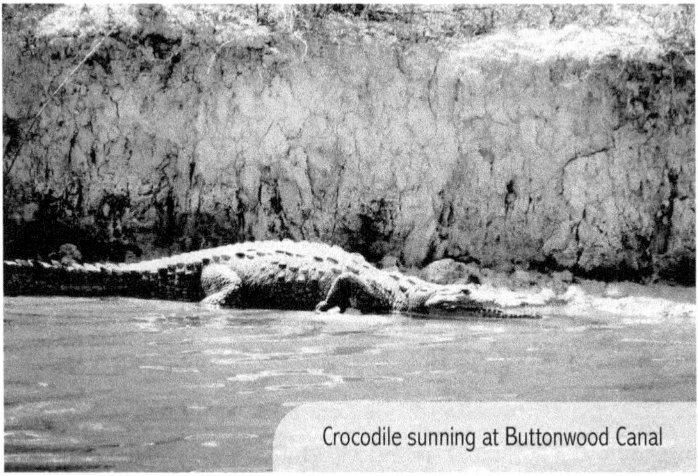
Crocodile sunning at Buttonwood Canal

roots arching into the water and their aerial roots hanging down in front of your boat.

Once inside Mud Lake, pass a couple of small islands, and paddle southwest and then south across the lake. Navigating is easy, for the trail is marked frequently with white PVC pipes. Mud Lake is a lovely, isolated spot that attracts a wide variety of birds. Look for roseate spoonbills roosting in the trees or sweeping their bills while feeding on the shore. Snowy egrets dot the trees, and anhingas and pelicans rest on snags as great blue and tricolored herons come and go.

At the southwest end of the lake, the passage to Bear Lake is marked with a PVC pipe. This channel ends at the Bear Lake Canoe Trail (see page 159), an old canal that originally ran east to west from the Buttonwood Canal out to Cape Sable. (This passage is no longer open all the way to Cape Sable.)

Turn right (west) and follow the Bear Lake Canoe Trail a few yards until it opens up at Bear Lake, where you might choose to step out of your boat onto the small beach. You will be standing on land that was deposited when the old Homestead Canal was dredged.

After exploring a bit on that land or paddling out into Bear Lake, turn around and head back the way you came, being sure not to miss the left turn into the passage to Mud Lake. Paddle east and then northeast across Mud Lake, through Mud Lake Creek, and then southeast down Coot Bay to U.S. Coast Guard (USCG) markers 2 and 1 (painted on a green floating barrel). Turn south and paddle the Buttonwood Canal back to the Flamingo Marina.

▶ **The Route: Option 2, via Coot Bay Pond** If you prefer not to paddle the straight 2-mile-long Buttonwood Canal, you can choose to put in at Coot Bay Pond. Marked by an NPS sign and a couple of picnic tables, this launch site is 3 miles up the park road from Flamingo (36 miles from the park entrance near Homestead).

Leave your vehicle at the side of the park road and launch from one of the two cleared areas on the banks of Coot Bay Pond. Paddle northwest across this small pond and enter the short channel that leads into Coot Bay. Once in the bay, paddle southwest toward USCG marker 2. Cross the entrance to the Buttonwood Canal on your left (southwest), and continue northwest along the shoreline of Coot Bay until you come to a NO MOTORS sign and Mud Lake Creek. Take this channel, marking the entry to a place where motorboaters are prohibited. It leads to areas that give you a sense of the wilderness while you are still close to the activity at Flamingo.

Once in Mud Lake, pass two small islands and head southwest and then west, following the white PVC pipes while watching the birds that seem to like roosting and feeding in these waters.

You might see ospreys, snowy egrets, cormorants, anhingas, pelicans, and pink roseate spoonbills. At the extreme southwest tip of the lake, you will enter the channel that ends at the Bear Lake Canoe Trail. Turn right (west) and paddle the short distance to the opening to Bear Lake. You might choose to paddle out into Bear Lake and do a bit of exploring, or step out at one of the open places on the south side of the Bear Lake Canoe Trail to walk along the bank that was created with the digging of the Homestead Canal in the early 1900s.

To return, paddle east for a short distance along the Bear Lake Canoe Trail until the passage to Mud Lake branches off to the left (north), and take that passage back into the lake. Follow the PVC pipes across Mud Lake and return to Coot Bay through Mud Lake Creek.

Travel southeast along the shoreline of Coot Bay and cross the entrance to the Buttonwood Canal near USCG marker 2. Paddle northeast across Coot Bay, keeping the expanse of the bay to your left (north). Continue along the shore, passing a cluster of wooden posts near the shoreline. You will shortly spot a NO MOTORS sign and a white PVC pipe on your right, marking the hard-to-spot entrance to Coot Bay Pond. Travel this short channel and cross the pond to the takeout.

▶ The Route: Option 3, via the Bear Lake Canoe Trail

Read the Bear Lake Canoe Trail description above and on page 159 for more information on access to this launch site and for a more thorough description of the trail. You will access the Bear Lake Canoe Trail put-in either from the access road or from the dock 2 miles up the Buttonwood Canal.

Launch your boat from the Bear Lake Canoe Trail dock, and paddle west down the trail channel, formerly known as the Homestead Canal. It was dredged in the 1920s to open up Cape Sable for development and was recently cleared again by a group of determined volunteers. You will pass an old Calusa shell mound about 1 mile along the canal, where the waterway dips in a gentle

U to the south. At 1.5 miles, the passage to Mud Lake comes in on the right (north) near white PVC pipes. (At this point you might choose to paddle a bit farther west to see Bear Lake before returning to this passage to Mud Lake.)

To proceed to Mud Lake, turn right into this channel, which opens into the lake. Paddle east and then northeast across lovely Mud Lake, following the white PVC pipes and watching for all the birds that benefit from these waters—ospreys, anhingas, cormorants, pelicans, snowy egrets, tricolored and blue herons, and pink roseate spoonbills.

Pass two small islands at the northeast end of Mud Lake, and enter mangrove-lined Mud Lake Creek, which leads to Coot Bay. Once in Coot Bay, turn right (east) and paddle along the shoreline of Coot Bay until you reach the entrance to Buttonwood Canal, indicated by USCG markers 1 and 2. Turn right (south) into Buttonwood Canal.

If your car is parked at Bear Lake Canoe Trail Dock, paddle approximately 0.5 mile to the dock on your right (west). Pull out on the dock, and portage along the path leading *left,* 250 feet to the parking area where you began your trip.

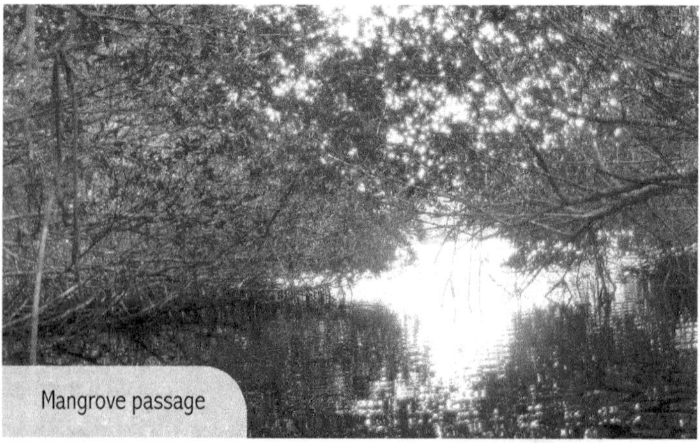

Mangrove passage

If you launched from the Flamingo Marina, continue paddling down the Buttonwood Canal to your takeout.

NINE MILE POND

NINE MILE POND

Distance: 5.2-mile loop

Paddle Time: 3–4 hours

Hazards: Low water levels February–May (check conditions at the visitor center)

Put-in on park road: N25° 15.234' W80° 47.866'

NPS marker 1: N25° 15.257' W80° 47.625'

NPS marker 44 (shortcut): N25° 15.426' W80° 46.770'

NPS marker 82 (end of shortcut): N25° 15.579' W80° 46.723'

Return entrance to Nine Mile Pond: N25° 15.311' W80° 47.776'

Maps & Charts: National Geographic Everglades TopoMap; trail guide available at the Flamingo VC or **nps.gov/ever/planyourvisit.**

▶ **Description** Don't let the name deceive you. The Nine Mile Pond Canoe Trail is just a bit more than 5 miles long, and you can even trim this distance by taking a shortcut, giving you a 3.5-mile paddle. Although you might run into waves on Nine Mile Pond itself if the day is windy, the rest of the trail is somewhat protected; it leads through mangrove tunnels and across sawgrass prairie.

Park your car at the Nine Mile Pond site, at the east side of the park road, 27 miles from the Ernest F. Coe Visitor Center at the park entrance (about 12 miles from the end of the road at Flamingo).

The name Nine Mile comes from the distance between Nine Mile Pond and the original NPS ranger station that once stood on Coot Bay Pond. The concessionaire at the Flamingo Marina rents the canoes that are stacked in the Nine Mile Pond parking area.

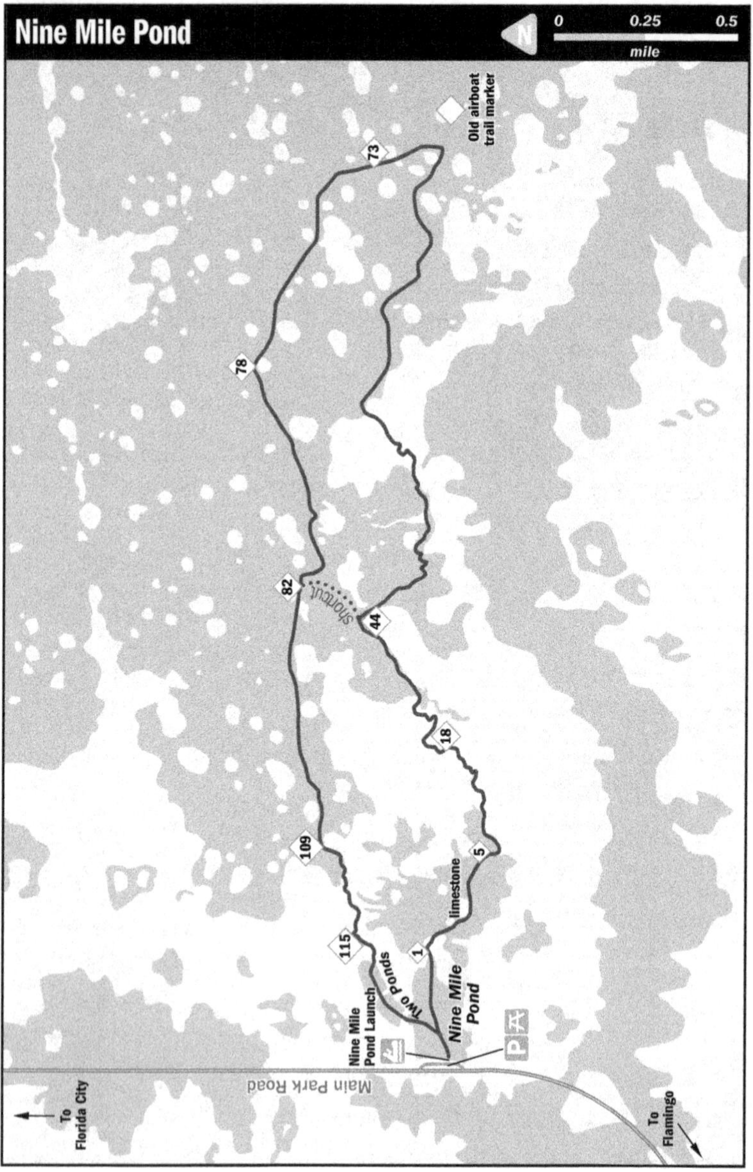
Nine Mile Pond
N
0
0.25
0.5
mile
Old airboat trail marker
73
78
82
Shortcut
44
18
109
5
limestone
115
1
Two ponds
Nine Mile Pond
Nine Mile Pond Launch
Main Park Road
To Florida City
To Flamingo

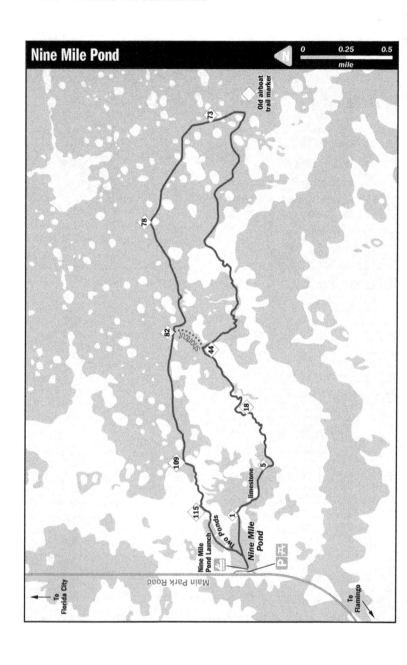

▶ **Route** The canoe trail is marked with more than 115 sequentially numbered PVC pipes. From the launch site, you will see marker 1 east across Nine Mile Pond itself. The first portion of your paddle passes marker 3 through red mangroves with their distinctive prop roots, as well as through cocoplums and buttonwoods. Soon the trail opens onto sawgrass prairie dotted with mangrove islands.

Note: The last time we paddled here, we ran into only one tricky spot, at marker 5, which was hidden by mangroves. Mangroves have a habit of growing. Any time you can't spot your marker, look in the edges of vegetation to see if it has been obscured by plant growth.

Near marker 6 you will begin to see white patches that look like sand under the water. Tap them with your paddle and you will discover that they are hard, the limestone bedrock (see page 253) of the Everglades.

Across from marker 12, you can see wax myrtle and a few Paurotis palms. Near marker 18 sits a larger group of slim

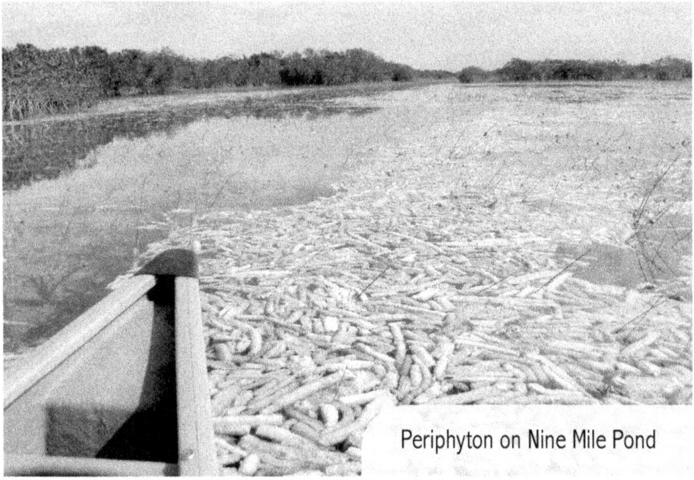

Periphyton on Nine Mile Pond

Paurotis palms that grow in clumps and are found in the wild only in Everglades National Park.

When you are close to the mangrove islands, you might see clusters of tiny white balls on emergent vegetation, just above the water line. These are the eggs of apple snails, the favorite food source of the endangered Everglades snail kite.

Around marker 19 you may spot a carnivorous air plant, the powdery Catopsis, with its yellow-flowered stalk and aloelike leaves. At marker 44 you will come to the shortcut mentioned above. If you choose this option, turn left (northeast) where you see the PVC pipes marked SHORTCUT. Paddle across the wet prairie to marker 82.

Continuing on the longer trail, you will pass Paurotis palms to the left at marker 52 and to the right at marker 59 and will continue to spot them along the way. Your paddles will rattle against spike rush as you cross the marsh, and you will see the bizarre formation called periphyton, a mass of algae, bacteria, microbes, and detritus that forms on and around solid submerged surfaces. Sometimes the periphyton looks like soft sheets of shale; other times it looks like breadsticks (the park brochure's description) or like floating beige spongy tops of cattails. Periphyton is essential to the ecology of the Everglades in that it holds water during the dry season, offering safe harbor for fish and insect eggs that will hatch when the rainy season comes again.

Also look for bladderwort, a tiny carnivorous water plant with yellow or pink flowers, and watch the fish swim in the shallow water under your boat.

From markers 93 to 100, the canoe trail follows an old airboat path. You are close to the takeout, but you will pass through two small ponds before returning to Nine Mile Pond. These two ponds are great sites for wildlife viewing. You may see wood storks, anhingas, and cormorants roosting in the mangroves that surround the pond, as well as alligators and crocodiles sunning themselves on muddy pullouts on the edge of the water.

When you reenter Nine Mile Pond, where you began the loop, turn right (west) to return to your takeout and your car.

NOBLE HAMMOCK CANOE TRAIL

NOBLE HAMMOCK CANOE TRAIL

Distance: 2-mile loop

Paddle Time: 2–3 hours

Hazards: Low water levels February–May (check conditions at the visitor center); heavy mosquitoes in the wet season; tight, twisting paddle through mangroves

Put-in on park road: N25° 14.135' W80° 49.072'

Noble Hammock: N25° 13.673' W80° 49.039'

Maps & Charts: USGS Quadrangle *West Lake, FL* 7.5-minute; National Geographic Everglades TopoMap

▶ **Description** Noble Hammock sounds like an easy trip—just 2 miles, out of the wind, and well-marked. But paddling this trail is a challenge, with a passage often so narrow that kayakers who can't take their paddles apart may have some difficulty steering in the narrow channels. Long kayaks and canoes will need to be carefully maneuvered through the tight turns, so have patience with your paddling companion as you repeatedly bump into mangroves.

The NPS has marked this route with more than 124 white PVC pipes, a good thing because navigating without the posts would be a nightmare. This tangled trail is called Noble Hammock after a hidden bit of high ground where, according to frontiersman Glen Simmons in his memoir, *Gladesmen*, Bill Noble, a storeowner in Homestead, ran a whiskey still during Prohibition.

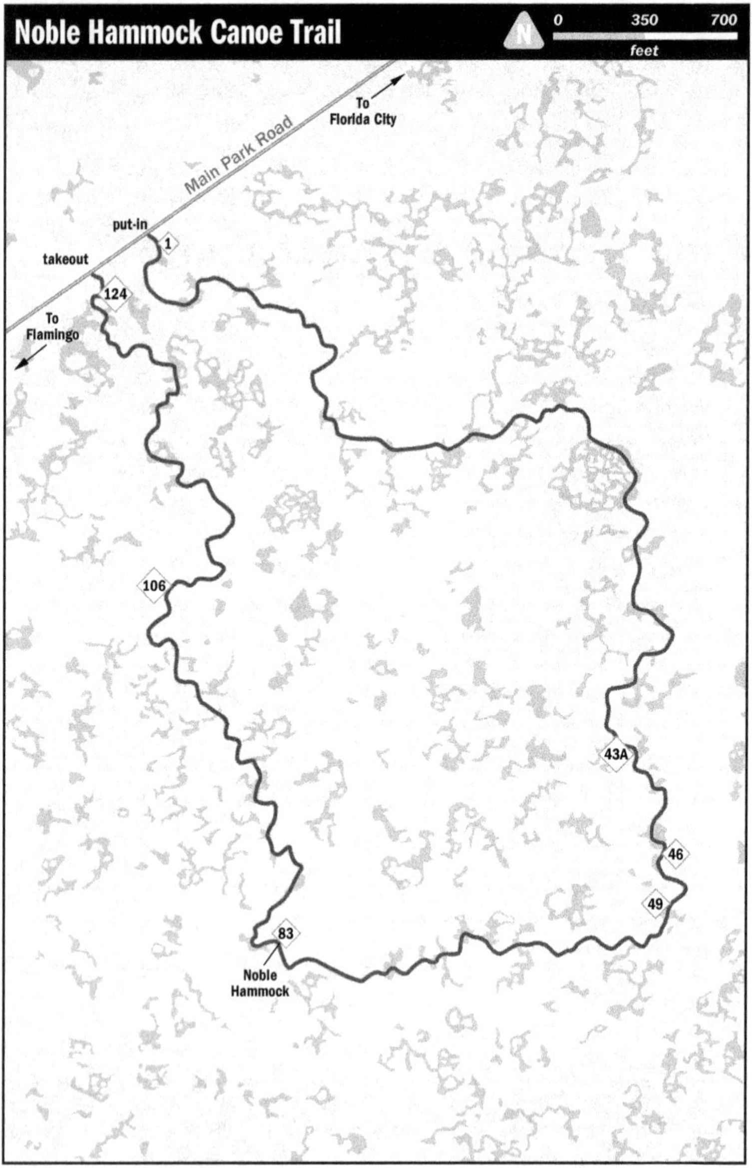
Noble Hammock Canoe Trail
N
0
350
700
feet
To
Florida City
Main Park Road
put-in
1
takeout
124
To
Flamingo
106
43A
46
49
83
Noble
Hammock

▶ **Route** Park on the permeable paving at the side of the park road. (Your takeout will be 100 yards southwest down the road.) The small dock where you will launch is 10 miles from Flamingo, 29 miles from the Ernest F. Coe Visitor Center. A poisonwood tree sits to the left of the launch site. This tree can be identified by the black spots on its oval leaves. It produces a rash similar to poison ivy, so don't touch it.

After you launch into the channel between red mangroves and buttonwoods, marker 1 will appear shortly on your right. Watch carefully for the markers—every time you think the trail goes left, it goes right, and every time you are positive that you should turn right, the trail veers left.

The vegetation throughout is lush with air plants, water plants, and areas of sawgrass. You will see the large, yellow-flowered carnivorous air plant, powdery Catopsis, and the yellow ropes of the leafless wormvine orchid.

At marker 46 you will see Paurotis palms and, near marker 49, the parasitic and invasive native plant called love vine or devil's gut that spreads its slender tendrils over and into its host.

Shortly after marker 83 you will arrive at Noble Hammock (see "Hammock," on page 251), marked with an NPS sign. Pull up and step out if you wish to explore the thick tangle of growth that hides the remnants of Bill Noble's still. As always, watch for snakes when you venture into overgrown vegetation. The canoe trail continues to marker 124 and the pullout on the park road. Your vehicle will be about 100 yards to your right.

OVERNIGHT PADDLES—FLAMINGO AREA

HELLS BAY CANOE TRAIL

HELLS BAY CANOE TRAIL

Distance: 3 miles one-way to Lard Can Campsite; 3.5 miles one-way to Pearl Bay Chickee; 5.5 miles one-way to Hells Bay Chickee

Paddle Time: 3.5 hours to Lard Can Campsite; 4 hours to Pearl Bay Chickee; 4.5 hours to Hells Bay Chickee

Hazards: Twisty, confusing channels through mangroves; heavy mosquitoes in the wet season; low water levels February–May (check conditions at the visitor center); Lard Can Campsite can be muddy and may be flooded in high water (check conditions at the visitor center)

Put-in on park road: N25° 13.952' W80° 49.397'

Lard Can Campsite: N25° 14.955' W80° 50.829'

Pearl Bay Chickee: N25° 15.573' W80° 51.375'

Hells Bay Chickee: N25° 15.195' W80° 52.708'

Maps & Charts: USGS Quadrangles *Mahogany Noble Hammock, FL* 7.5-minute, *West Lake, FL* 7.5-minute; NOAA Nautical Chart 11433 (useful from Lard Can to Hells Bay); Waterproof Chart 39 (useful from Lard Can to Hells Bay); National Geographic Everglades TopoMap; trail map available at the Flamingo VC or **nps.gov/ever/planyourvisit.**

▶ **Description** Designated a National Recreation Trail, this beautiful but twisty paddle is aptly described as "Hell to get into, and Hell to get out of." Author Larry Perez, in his *Words on the Wilderness*, credits Barney Parker, the first ranger in Everglades National Park, for coining this phrase.

As you maneuver through the mangrove tangle along the first 3 miles of the Hells Bay Canoe Trail, charts and maps and GPS won't help; you'll be thankful for the more than 180 white PVC pipes the NPS has used to mark the channel. Glen Simmons, in his memoir, *Gladesmen*, describes it this way: "This trail twisted and turned worser than any snake and was grown thick

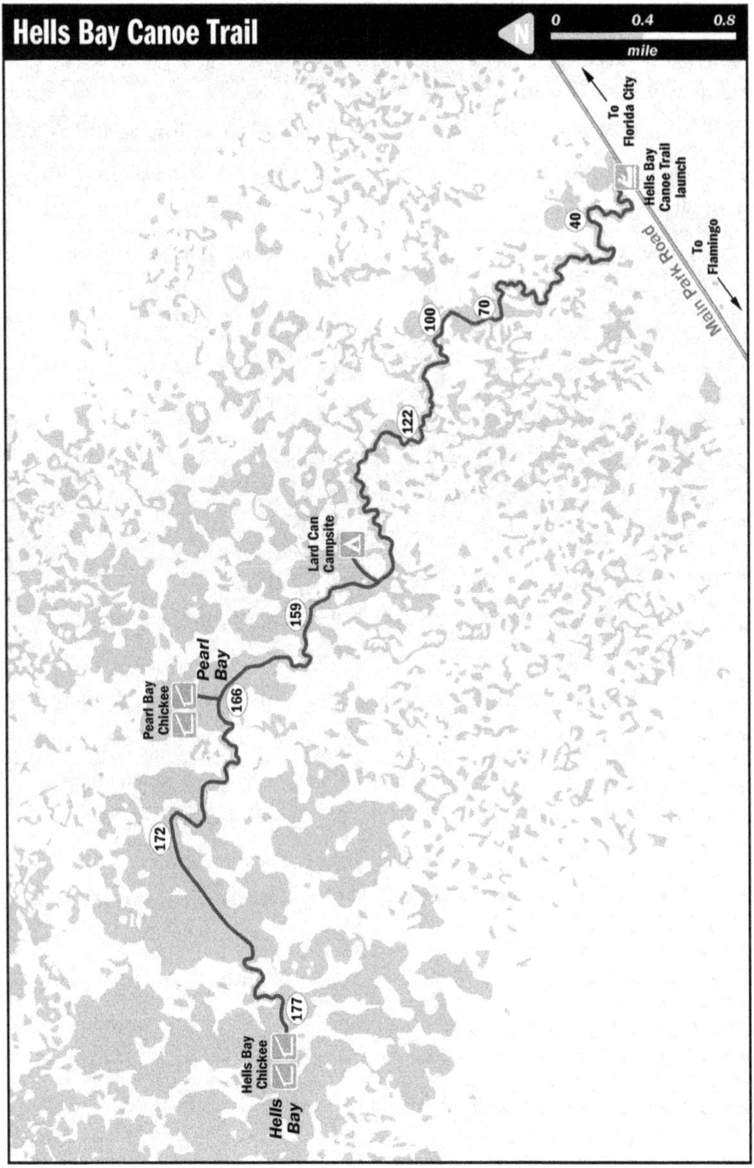

Hells Bay Canoe Trail

with mangroves." Paddling this channel will give you an understanding of how hard-to-follow routes such as these were ideal for moonshiners and gator hunters.

But this paddle has its interesting attributes: Importantly, it gives you a close-up view of the mangrove ecosystem. In addition to the red mangroves that line the channel, see the cocoplums, wax myrtles, buttonwoods, ferns, and sawgrass that grow here. If you paddle in the winter, you won't see the summertime blossoms of the orchids growing along the waterway, but you can hunt for the small, slender leaves of the dollar orchids and can easily spot the ropy yellow-green "trunks" of the leafless wormvine orchid. Unlike the orchids, powdery Catopsis, a carnivorous bromeliad, displays its stalks of yellow flowers in the wintertime.

En route to Hells Bay, you will be able to visit and possibly camp at Lard Can, one of the few dry spots in the area. It has been inhabited over the years by Calusa, Seminoles, and early Florida pioneers.

However, Lard Can is often soggy and underwater. Check with the Flamingo VC for current conditions. Or you can spend the night on Pearl Bay Chickee, the only handicap-accessible chickee in Everglades National Park, or at Hells Bay Chickee, which lies 2 miles beyond Pearl Bay. It is your choice whether to paddle into this area and return the same day or camp for the night in the backcountry.

If you plan to stay at Lard Can Campsite (see page 229), Pearl Bay Chickee (see page 232), or Hells Bay Chickee (see page 222), remember to make the required reservations in person at the visitor center within 24 hours of your overnight date.

▶ **Route** This is a good paddling route on windy days because much of the trail is sheltered in the mangrove passages. However, avoid this trip in the summer, as the mosquitoes can be unbearable. Kayakers with two-piece paddles may want to take them apart to make the turns a bit easier.

Park your car on the north side of the park road 10 miles from Flamingo (29 miles from the Ernest F. Coe Visitor Center) at the Hells Bay Canoe Trail put-in, where you will find a small dock.

The trail is closed to motorboaters from the put-in on the park road to Lard Can, where it opens up onto the first bay in a series.

You will immediately paddle into a red mangrove tangle; the mangroves are short here because the soil is thin over the limestone bedrock and the water is brackish. Follow the white PVC pipes that mark the trail; they are numbered sequentially starting at the put-in and ending at marker 177 at Hells Bay Chickee. Note that the numbers on the pipes are often easier to read from the direction opposite the way you are traveling and that the numbers are sometimes obliterated by the weather. If you paddle for a while and don't see a marker, turn around and retrace your path, as you don't want to become lost in this maze of mangrove islands.

You will come to a small, dry spot shortly after marker 45 and another dry area just before marker 80. Both places give you a chance to step out and take a break. Look for Paurotis palms before marker 70 and at marker 114. With slender trunks and silvery-green leaves, Paurotis palms grow wild only in Everglades National Park.

Three miles into the paddle, the channel opens onto a bay. From this point on you will be able to use your navigational charts, although you can continue to follow the PVC pipes all the way to Hells Bay Chickee. At marker 155, as you enter this bay, look to the right (northeast), and about 100 yards away you will spot a white pipe that marks the Lard Can Campsite. Even if you have not made reservations to spend the night, paddle over to take a look.

Because it is one of the few dry spots in this part of the Everglades, Lard Can is full of human history. In addition to the early Calusa and the later Seminoles, this campsite was a base for Florida pioneers and gator hunters. Lard Can takes its name from the tin pails with tight lids that pioneers used to store their food, clothing, and supplies when they ventured into the interior. Often they buried their lard can "suitcases" to keep them safe between trips, and they also turned lard cans into freshwater distillers when they had to spend weeks in brackish environments.

From Lard Can, follow the PVC markers along the western shore of the bay and turn west and then north into the channels that lead to Pearl Bay. Now that you are in open water, you might have to contend with wind and waves, but it will be a welcome break from the tight paddling of the mangrove maze. Look for ospreys flying, or watch for a bald eagle perched on a dead tree. You may see rafts of coot—those small, black ducklike birds with thick white bills—on the water (see page 249).

Pearl Bay Chickee lies directly north across the bay near marker 166, tucked close to the mangrove shoreline. If you plan to continue 2 more miles to Hells Bay, follow the PVC pipes west, as they lead out of Pearl Bay into a channel that opens into a small bay. The trail leads northwest through this small bay and then southwest through a larger bay into the channel that takes you into Hells Bay. Once in the bay you will see Hells Bay Chickee near marker 177.

Return the way you came, following the markers in descending numerical order to your takeout on the park road.

Note: It is possible to reach Whitewater Bay and ultimately Flamingo from Hells Bay Chickee by taking the East River, but only experienced navigators and paddlers should try it. There are no markers beyond the chickee. You are dependent upon chart and compass from that point on, and Whitewater Bay can be rough with waves. Then, once you arrive at Flamingo, you will have to shuttle the 10 miles back to the put-in on the park road.

JOHNSON KEY

JOHNSON KEY

Distance: 8.5 miles one-way

Paddle Time: 4 hours

Hazards: Powerboats along the route; wind and waves; shallow water in Florida Bay

Flamingo Marina: N25° 08.541' W80° 55.394'

Entrance to Flamingo Marina and USCG marker 18: N25° 08.458' W80° 55.330'

Murray Key: N25° 06.542' W80° 56.602'

Intersection with Conchie Channel: N25° 05.430' W80° 56.303'

Clive Key: N25° 04.826' W80° 55.927'

Johnson Key Chickee: N25° 03.073' W80° 54.427'

Maps & Charts: Waterproof Chart 33E (Florida Bay); NOAA Nautical Chart 11451

▶ **Description** Southernmost of all the paddles in this guidebook, this route takes you out into the shallow, island-dotted expanse of Florida Bay. Here you can expect to see an abundance of birds—gulls, terns, and cormorants perching on channel markers; pelicans and cormorants diving for fish; and ibis, egrets, and herons roosting on the mangrove islands or wading in the flats. Watch for sharks, dolphins, fish, rays, crabs, and other sea life as you paddle these shallow waters.

Your destination is Johnson Key Chickee, perched high over the seagrass beds in Florida Bay.

Optimal time to launch is near high tide, when water levels are at their highest. Even though you can spot the chickee in

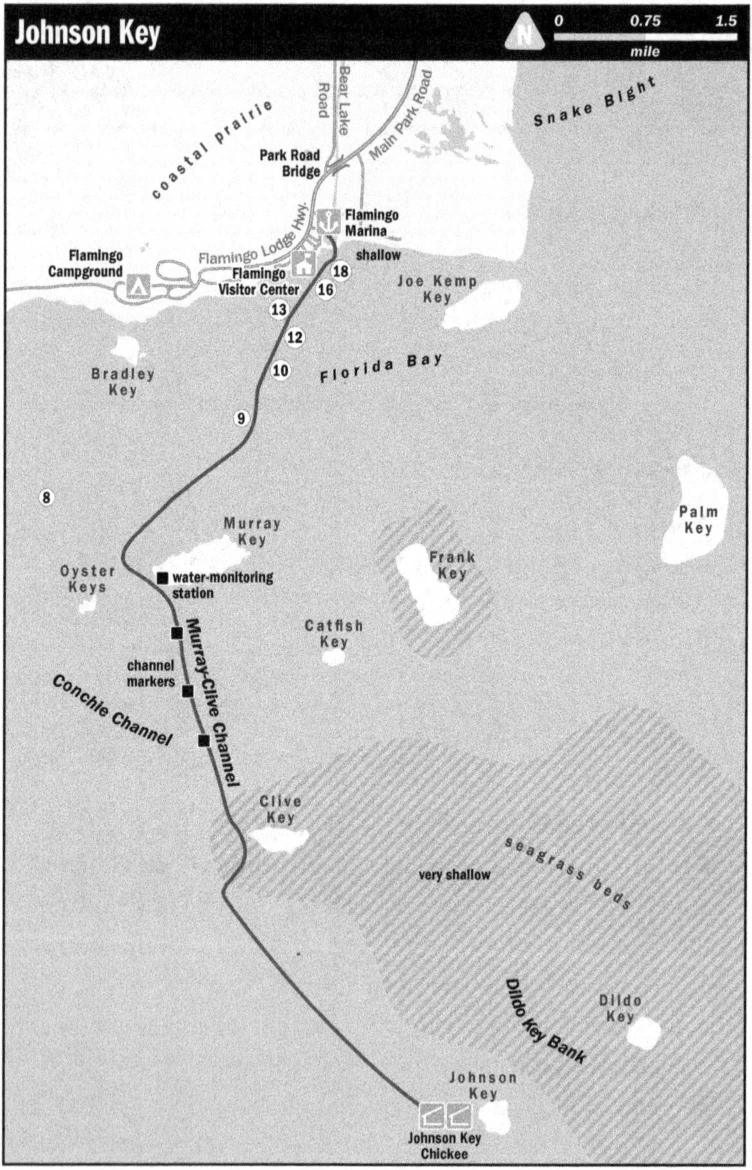
Johnson Key
0
0.75
1.5
mile
Snake Bight
Bear Lake Road
Main Park Road
coastal prairie
Park Road Bridge
Flamingo Marina
Flamingo Lodge Hwy.
shallow
Flamingo Campground
Flamingo Visitor Center
18
16
13
12
10
9
8
Joe Kemp Key
Bradley Key
Florida Bay
Palm Key
Murray Key
Frank Key
Oyster Keys
water-monitoring station
Catfish Key
channel markers
Murray-Clive Channel
Conchie Channel
Clive Key
seagrass beds
very shallow
Dildo Key Bank
Dildo Key
Johnson Key
Johnson Key Chickee

the distance when you stand on the deck of the Flamingo VC, don't be tempted to paddle directly there. As author Ted Levin writes in *Liquid Land*, "Except for a fish or a porpoise at high tide nothing crosses Florida Bay in a straight line." Rather, follow the marked Murray-Clive Channel to avoid getting stuck on the banks and damaging the seagrass beds.

▶ **Route** Put in at the boat launch at the Florida Bay side of the Flamingo Marina, and travel south, following USCG markers 18 to 9, then southwest toward USCG marker 8. You will spot the marked Murray-Clive Channel at the west side of Murray Key.

Pass between Murray Key, with its water-monitoring station, and the smaller Oyster Keys to the west. The Oyster Keys are the site of an important event in Everglades history: On Saturday morning, July 8, 1905, Guy Bradley, game warden in the Everglades, was shot and killed as he confronted plumers in the act of shooting "a mess of birds" in the Oyster Keys rookery. The man who confessed to killing Bradley was freed by a jury that looked unfavorably on new game laws that prohibited such wildlife destruction. Bradley's neighbors, however, burned down the murderer's Flamingo home. (The quote and details of this event were gathered from interviews with Bradley's family that are recounted in Stuart McIver's book *Death in the Everglades*.)

To continue, follow the Murray-Clive Channel south. (Conchie Channel bears off to the west.) Once you pass Clive Key (in nesting season you can both see and hear the birds that use this key as a rookery), you will spy the Johnson Key Chickee in the distance, looking very much like a boat out on the water. Travel southeast toward the chickee, which lies between Johnson Key on the left (east) and the larger Man of War Key in the distance on the right (west). (Due to our map scale, Man of War Key is not shown on our Johnson Key map, on the opposite page.)

Once at the chickee, pull into one of the two boat slips. This chickee is high off the water (see the Johnson Key Chickee description, on page 227), so you may struggle to lift your gear onto the platform, but once you climb up, you will realize just what an outstanding panorama this campsite offers.

Return to Flamingo by the same route in reverse. When you see the radio tower, you may be tempted to paddle directly toward Flamingo because it would appear to be a direct route.

Tern on Florida Bay channel marker

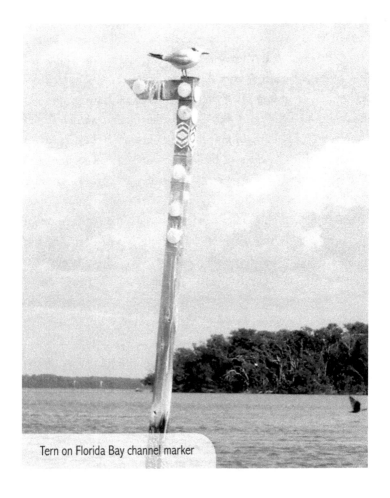

But please do not succumb to this inclination because the shallows of Dildo Key Bank lie directly in your path. (Dildo Key, by the way, is named for certain members of the Cactaceae, or cactus, family.) Instead, head to the western (left) side of Clive Key before picking up the Murray-Clive Channel. Pass to the left (west) of Murray Key, and turn northeast toward the USCG markers that lead you back to the marina.

SHARK POINT

SHARK POINT

Distance: 9.5 miles one-way

Paddle Time: 4 hours

Hazards: Shallow water in Florida Bay; powerboats along the route; potential wind and waves

Flamingo Marina: N25° 08.541' W80° 55.394'

Entrance to Flamingo canal and USCG marker 18: N25° 08.458' W80° 55.330'

Joe Kemp Key: N25° 07.899' W80° 54.587'

Joe Kemp Channel: N25° 07.770' W80° 54.080'

Tin Can Channel: N25° 07.522' W80° 53.285'

Buoy Key: N25° 07.308' W80° 49.973'

Shark Point Chickee: N25° 08.469' W80° 48.147'

Maps & Charts: Waterproof Chart 33E (Florida Bay) or 39; NOAA Nautical Chart 11433

▶ **Description** If this is your first visit to Flamingo, you might gaze out across Florida Bay and assume that it's a deep, easy-to-paddle body of water. Never assume. For helpful information on "reading" Florida Bay, be sure to pick up the NPS brochure "Florida Bay Map and Guide," which quotes guide Rusty Albury: "Outside the channels, everything's shallow." Also, this route is not one for a windy day. Although Florida Bay itself is shallow, it can produce dangerous waves.

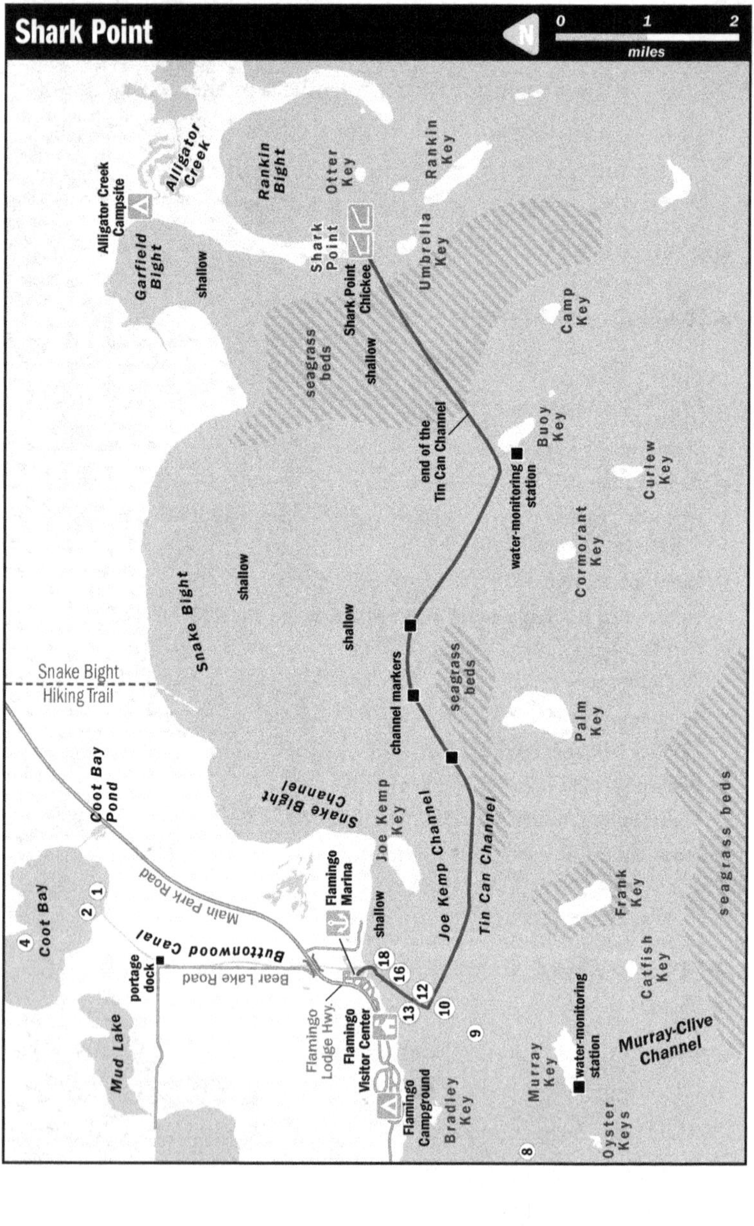
Shark Point
N
0
1
2
miles
Alligator Creek Campsite
Alligator Creek
Rankin Bight
Otter Key
Rankin Key
Garfield Bight
shallow
Shark Point
Shark Point Chickee
Umbrella Key
seagrass beds
shallow
Camp Key
end of the Tin Can Channel
Buoy Key
water-monitoring station
Curlew Key
Cormorant Key
Snake Bight
shallow
shallow
Snake Bight Hiking Trail
channel markers
seagrass beds
Palm Key
Coot Bay Pond
Snake Bight Channel
Joe Kemp Key
Joe Kemp Channel
Tin Can Channel
seagrass beds
Coot Bay
Main Park Road
Flamingo Marina
shallow
Frank Key
Buttonwood Canal
portage dock
Bear Lake Road
Catfish Key
Mud Lake
Flamingo Lodge Hwy.
Flamingo Visitor Center
water-monitoring station
Murray-Clive Channel
Murray Key
Flamingo Campground
Bradley Key
Oyster Keys
1
2
4
8
9
10
12
13
16
18

The beauty of this shallow water is that sunlight easily reaches the sparkling, emerald-green seagrass beds, home to an abundance of sea creatures. Often barely inches deep, these waters are also a feeding ground for a multitude of wading birds, such as egrets, herons, and roseate spoonbills.

Florida Bay also is a fisherman's paradise, and motorboaters will be your constant companions as you travel the Tin Can Channel, the only deep passage across this portion of Florida Bay. The Tin Can Channel is marked on both sides with tall wooden posts, with directional arrows that point to the center of the passage. The powerboats come at great speed, so when they pass, stay just outside, north or south of the markers.

▶ **Route** Launch from the Flamingo Marina and pass USCG marker 18 as you enter Florida Bay. Paddle southwest past the two small islands that lie just outside the marina channel. Do not be tempted to turn immediately east—the water here is extremely

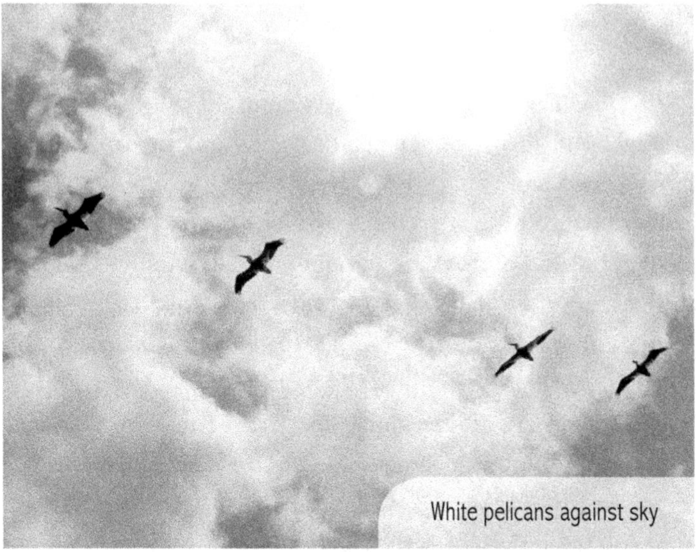

White pelicans against sky

shallow. Rather, continue southwest until you have sufficient water depth to head southeast toward the wooden posts that mark both Joe Kemp Channel and Tin Can Channel. Use your navigational charts, which clearly show water depth.

Particularly at low tide, in order to be certain that you are in deep-enough water, continue southwest until you reach USCG marker 12 before making the turn east.

Note: Be aware that even though the water is shallow, the mud may be extremely deep. If you do get stuck, do not step out of your boat. Wait for high tide.

Once you are headed east, pass large Joe Kemp Key to your left (north). After the key, the marked Joe Kemp Channel branches off to the left (north) and leads into the Snake Bight Channel.

Do not go there. Instead, note the markers lying before you, heading east, that indicate the Tin Can Channel. You will follow the length of this channel. To your left, the flats of Snake Bight are feeding grounds for great egrets that look remarkably like sailboats in the distance. (You might hike the Snake Bight Hiking Trail when you return to Flamingo and see the bight from the land side.)

The Tin Can Channel curves northeast past Palm Key on the right and then dips southeast toward Cormorant Key (also on the right) and then to Buoy Key. You can see motorboaters in the distance as they travel this passage. Buoy Key is easy to identify because of the water-monitoring station on its near side and because the channel makes such a close approach. At this point, with binoculars, you can see Shark Point Chickee to the northeast (left).

Paddle past the remaining Tin Can Channel markers and head directly northeast across the bay. Don't be tempted to cut across the bay as soon as you see the chickee; stay in the channel until you reach the end of the channel markers.

Pull into one of the boat slips at the chickee. A wealth of life lies in the seagrass that sways in the current right below you: an array of fishes as well as marine invertebrates—spider crabs, sea urchins, and jellyfish—congregate in these meadows of vegetation. You might even spot a small shark swimming here, under Shark Point Chickee. For more on this rich underwater universe, see "Seagrass," on page 259.

To return, head southwest to Buoy Key and the eastern end of the Tin Can Channel. Take the Tin Can Channel to its western end near Flamingo and then follow the USCG markers into the marina. Again, do not take shortcuts. The water is very shallow around Joe Kemp Key.

SOUTH JOE RIVER

SOUTH JOE RIVER

Distance: 9 miles one-way

Paddle Time: 4 hours

Hazards: Powerboats all along the route; wind and waves on Coot Bay, Whitewater Bay, and the Joe River

Coot Bay Pond: N25° 10.966' W80° 53.884'

Entrance to Coot Bay from Coot Bay Pond: N25° 11.221' W80° 54.148'

Flamingo Marina: N25° 08.541' W80° 55.394'

USCG marker 2: N25° 11.102' W80° 54.726'

USCG marker 8: N25° 12.202' W80° 55.607'

USCG marker 10: N25° 12.708' W80° 55.857'

South channel to South Joe River Chickee: N25° 13.347' W81° 00.462'

South Joe River Chickee: N25° 13.320' W81° 00.641'

Maps & Charts: NOAA Nautical Chart 11433; Waterproof Chart 39

▶ **Description** This route gives you an opportunity to spend the night on a chickee in the backcountry. You will paddle across well-marked Coot Bay, touch the south end of massive Whitewater Bay, and follow a gradually narrowing Joe River to your overnight destination.

Note: We do not recommend this paddle for beginners, as the Joe River section of this paddle can be challenging. Be sure to check the weather and wind directions before you head out, both for the launch date and the date of return.

▶ **Route** Launch from the main park road at the Coot Bay Pond put-in, 4 miles northeast of Flamingo (and 34 miles southwest of the Ernest F. Coe Visitor Center). Paddle through a small opening in the mangroves at the edge of quiet Coot Bay Pond, and cross the pond in a northwesterly direction.

Exit through a short mangrove tunnel into broader Coot Bay, which may be as smooth as glass or a windy, strenuous paddle. (You can also enter Coot Bay by taking the Buttonwood Canal from the Flamingo Marina.)

Following USCG markers 3 to 8, paddle northwest. Depending on wind conditions, you may want to keep right and follow the shoreline until you come to Tarpon Creek. This creek meanders a bit and is usually calm, though at the changing of the tide you may find the current tugging either with you or against you. When you exit Tarpon Creek, you will be at the southern extremity of Whitewater Bay.

Turn left (west) at USCG marker 10 and paddle due west on the Joe River, which, at this point, is very wide. Be aware that this section of the paddle can be challenging when the wind is high.

As you continue paddling west, the river will eventually begin to narrow and turn, so your direction will shift southwest, and then northwest. You will paddle approximately 6 miles on the Joe River.

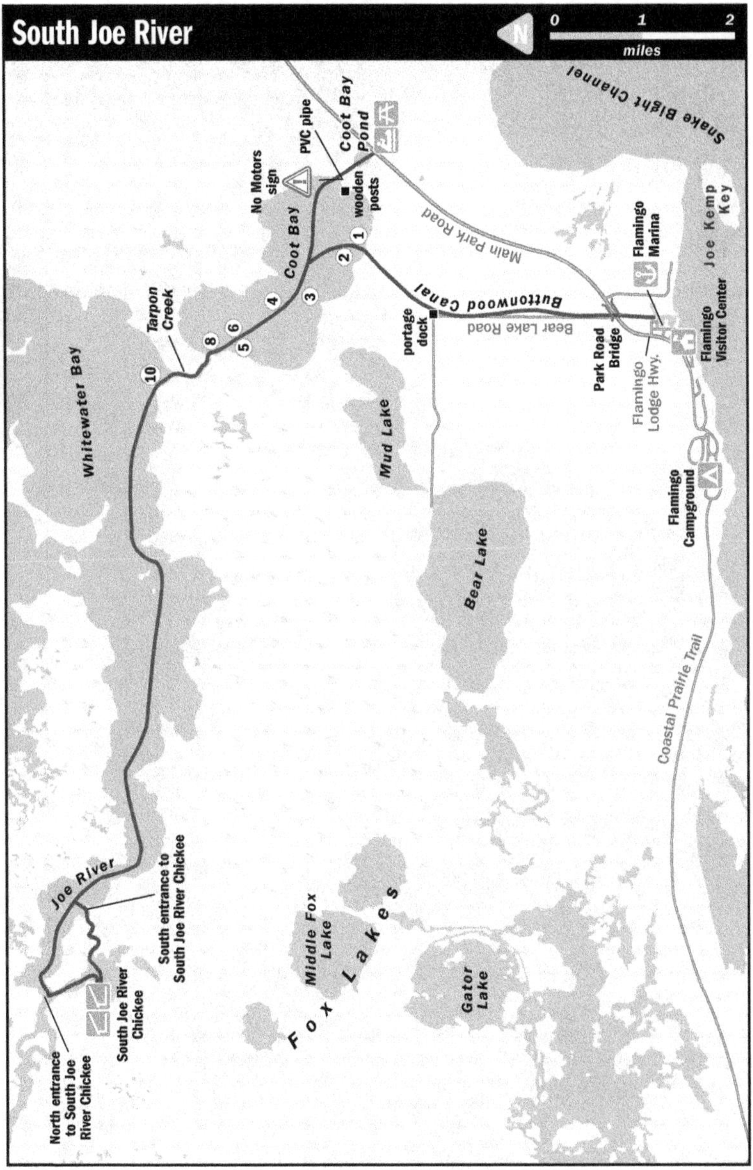
South Joe River
N
0
1
2
miles
Snake Bight Channel
Coot Bay Pond
PVC pipe
No Motors sign
wooden posts
Coot Bay
Main Park Road
Buttonwood Canal
Bear Lake Road
portage dock
Flamingo Marina
Joe Kemp Key
Flamingo Visitor Center
Park Road Bridge
Flamingo Lodge Hwy.
Tarpon Creek
Whitewater Bay
Mud Lake
Bear Lake
Flamingo Campground
Coastal Prairie Trail
Joe River
South entrance to South Joe River Chickee
South Joe River Chickee
North entrance to South Joe River Chickee
Middle Fox Lake
Fox Lakes
Gator Lake
1
2
3
4
5
6
8
10

Keep an eye on your navigational chart as you advance, watching for your cutoff channel on the left (southwest). When you see a MANATEE ZONE sign on your right, the entrance to the bay where the South Joe Chickee sits will appear shortly on your left (south). Take this channel, which will curve behind a large mangrove island, and arrive at the small bay where the South Joe River Chickee is perched, facing east. Because this chickee is behind an island, you will not be able to see it until you paddle behind that island. If you miss the first channel leading toward the chickee, you can pick up the one on the other side of the mangrove island and paddle southeast about 0.5 mile to the chickee.

There must be times when the wind isn't blowing at South Joe River Chickee, but we have not yet managed to land there at one of those times. We strongly recommend that you bungee or tie the four corners of your tent to the chickee posts, and place heavy objects in the four corners of the tent to hold it securely in place. (For a detailed description of the South Joe River Chickee, see page 238.)

The next day, after you have enjoyed the colors of the sun rising across the bay, listened to the morning birds, and perhaps watched an alligator or dolphin swim by, you will retrace your path.

Leaving the chickee, paddle across the small bay it overlooks and out through the channel by which you arrived, curving back around the mangrove island to the Joe River.

Turn right at the river and paddle southeast, later east, as the river widens. If you find that, in spite of planning and weather indications, you have a rough paddle on your hands, take advantage of occasional mangrove islands for taking shelter, drinking water, and resting a bit before moving on. Or, if it seems advisable, hug the right shoreline. At USCG marker 10, turn right (south) into Tarpon Creek, and then follow the USCG markers across Coot Bay until you see a cluster of poles near the shore to the left of USCG marker 2. The narrow, hard-to-spot passage to Coot Bay Pond lies just north of these wooden poles and is marked by a white PVC pipe and a No Motors sign. Cross Coot Bay Pond and take out where you put in.

For those of you whose paddle began from the Flamingo Marina and up the Buttonwood Canal, follow USCG markers 8 to 1 across Coot Bay Pond and enter the Buttonwood Canal at marker 1, a green buoy floating in the water. Paddle 3 miles back to the marina.

WEST LAKE TO ALLIGATOR CREEK

WEST LAKE TO ALLIGATOR CREEK

Distance: 8.5 miles one-way

Paddle Time: 5 hours

Hazards: Wind on West Lake and Long Lake; downed branches in the channels; potential for slippery marl landing at Alligator Creek; heavy mosquitoes at Alligator Creek Campsite

West Lake launch: N25° 12.878' W80° 51.017'

Exit from West Lake: N25° 12.057' W80° 48.107'

Long Lake: N25° 11.949' W80° 48.071'

Entrance to Mangrove Creek: N25° 11.235' W80° 46.438'

Entrance to the Lungs: N25° 10.830' W80° 46.240'

Entrance to Alligator Creek: N25° 10.330' W80° 46.624'

Alligator Creek Campsite: N25° 10.568' W80° 47.601'

Maps & Charts: USGS Quadrangle *West Lake, FL* 7.5-minute; NOAA Nautical Chart 11433; Waterproof Chart 39; National Geographic Everglades TopoMap

▶ **Description** Following the West Lake Canoe Trail, you will paddle through several lakes that are connected by narrow mangrove channels. The trail leads to Alligator Creek Campsite, near the spot where Alligator Creek empties into Garfield Bight off Florida Bay. This route will give you an experience in miniature of what paddling the 99-mile Wilderness Waterway is like. Depending on conditions, you might be paddling against wind and waves in the open water of the lakes; you will work your way through creeks overgrown by mangrove branches, much like the Waterway's Nightmare (see page 256); you will search for markers and can test your navigational skills by reading your charts; and you will experience a bit of the ambiguity of not being quite sure at times that you are on the trail.

For a simpler experience, you might choose to paddle out into West Lake and Long Lake and then head back, making this a day trip. We have seen kayakers with sails skimming along the water in West Lake, enjoying a windy day. But if you want to prevail for an overnight, read on.

▶ **Route** The put-in is off the park road at the West Lake parking area (7 miles northeast of Flamingo and 32 miles southwest of the park entrance near Homestead). At the West Lake parking area, you will find a hiking trail with an observation platform, restrooms, picnic tables under a pavilion, a launch, and four docks. After launching, paddle right (south) down the channel that leads to West Lake.

Once in the lake, travel west along its 3-mile length. The NPS brochures and the National Geographic TopoMap show the trail as following the south shoreline, but take wind conditions into consideration as you decide whether to follow the south or north shoreline or paddle directly down the center of the lake. The passage into Long Lake lies at the southeast end of West Lake and is marked by a white PVC pipe. From this point on, motors are not allowed, so you will soon get a sense of being out in the wilderness.

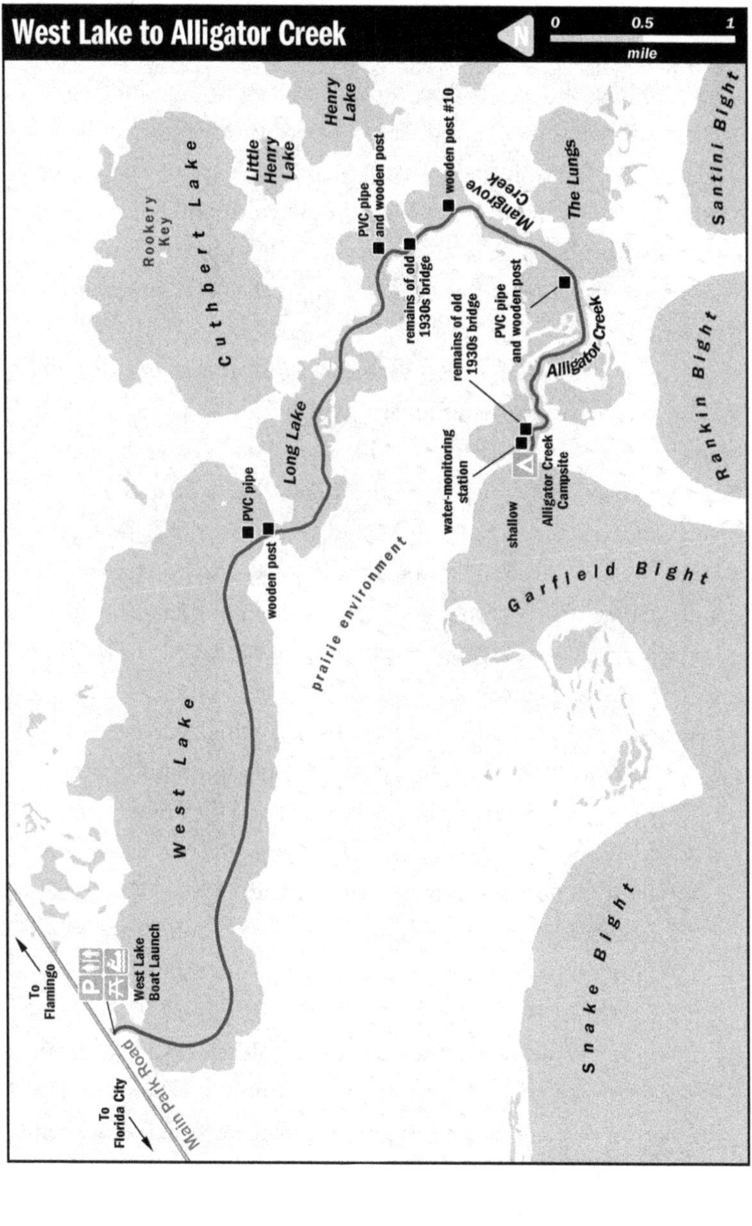
West Lake to Alligator Creek
N
0
0.5
1
mile
West Lake
Cuthbert Lake
Rookery Key
Little Henry Lake
Henry Lake
Long Lake
PVC pipe
wooden post
PVC pipe and wooden post
remains of old 1930s bridge
wooden post #10
Mangrove Creek
The Lungs
PVC pipe and wooden post
Alligator Creek
remains of old 1930s bridge
water-monitoring station
Alligator Creek Campsite
shallow
prairie environment
Garfield Bight
Rankin Bight
Santini Bight
Snake Bight
West Lake Boat Launch
To Flamingo
To Florida City
Main Park Road

The passage to Long Lake is canopied by mangroves, their prop roots encrusted with barnacles. When you emerge onto the lake, paddle east and then southeast across the 2-mile-long lake.

Again, the park brochure and National Geographic Topo-Map direct the paddler to follow the south shore of Long Lake, but take the winds into account. Choose your shoreline or down the middle. Check your charts, and you will observe that Cuthbert Lake lies to the northeast of Long Lake. For more on this historic lake, see page 249.

Paddle east and then southeast across the length of Long Lake, passing two series of islands. Watch for the occasional PVC pipe and/or older wooden poles that mark the route. At the eastern end of Long Lake you will see the white PVC pipe and wooden post that mark the entrance to Mangrove Creek. Paddle down this creek, which leads to The Lungs, a large bay shaped vaguely like human lungs. As they were along the route to Long Lake, the mangrove prop roots are encrusted with barnacles and look as if they are wearing socks. The passage is almost blocked in places by downed trees and branches. Much of the downed wood you see is big, twisty buttonwood, which resembles large pieces of driftwood.

The creek opens up into a wide area and then narrows again at wooden post 10, which is almost obscured by the mangroves. Continue paddling Mangrove Creek until it ends at The Lungs. Paddle south, leaving the expanse of The Lungs to the left (east).

A PVC pipe and wooden pole mark the entrance to Alligator Creek on your right (west). Follow the creek as it winds first west, then north, and then southwest. When Alligator Creek widens for a stretch, look for roseate spoonbills in the trees. On the narrower passages you might spot alligators and American crocodiles basking on the shore in the sun.

You will pass the wooden remnants of a bridge, the "cotton road," that crossed the creek back in the 1930s. At that time roads were constructed to get workers into the Glades to eradicate Florida tree cotton, which was thought to be infested with the pink bollworm and, therefore, a threat to native cotton.

You will pass a water-monitoring station on the right before reaching the Alligator Creek Campsite on the right (north) bank. Use caution as you pull up. Particularly at low tide and after rain, the takeout can be slippery with claylike marl.

For your return trip, launch into Alligator Creek and turn left (east), paddling back the way you came. Paddle the channel, watching for the PVC pipes and wooden posts that mark the route.

Once in The Lungs, turn left and paddle northeast as you watch for the PVC pipe that marks the narrowing of the Lungs and the passage into Mangrove Creek. The creek widens at wooden post 10 and then narrows again to the northwest at a PVC pipe and another wooden pole. In this stretch of Mangrove Creek, you might spot the wooden posts that remain from another bridge for an old roadway; it is marked by a dotted line on the 7.5-minute *Flamingo, FL* quadrant.

When Mangrove Creek opens onto the southeastern end of Long Lake, turn right (north) to reach the body of Long Lake. Watch for the PVC pipes and wooden posts. Paddle west and then northwest along this narrow end of Long Lake. Out in the main body of the lake, travel 2 miles northwest.

Watch for the wooden post that marks the passage that leads to West Lake. Paddle north along this passage and turn left (west) into West Lake. Paddle the 3-mile length of this lake to the PVC pipe and wooden post that mark the channel to the takeout at the West Lake parking area.

Note: From Alligator Creek, an alternative return trip (not shown on our map) would be to turn right from the Alligator Creek Campsite and paddle out into Garfield Bight, heading south into Florida Bay and then southwest toward Flamingo. Do not choose this option at low tide because you will get stuck in the shallow water of the bight. If you do paddle out with sufficient water, understand that you could also get stuck in shallow Snake Bight if you hug the shore on your way to Flamingo. A better choice when you enter Florida Bay would be to head out into the Tin Can Channel, indicated on Waterproof Chart 33B, and take that approach to Flamingo. Also realize that if you choose this option, you will need a shuttle to return to the West Lake launch from Flamingo.

Part Four:

Summer Paddling

Summer high tide

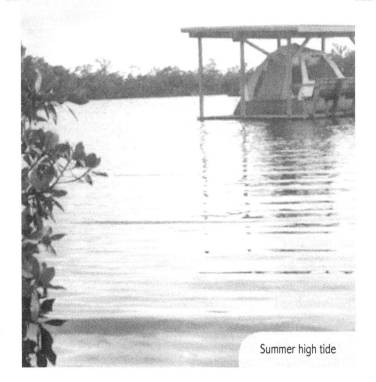

You'll hear a lot about why you shouldn't paddle the Everglades in summer: the heat, the no-see-ums, and those "swamp angels" known as mosquitoes. Well, we aren't going to deny that heat and insects are an issue in a South Florida summer, but we've done some great summer paddling in the areas north and south of the Everglades Wilderness Waterway and on parts of the 99-mile Waterway that are conducive to day and overnight paddles. If you'd like to give summer paddling a try, or if summer is your only opportunity to explore these areas, we would suggest that you read this section carefully.

Throughout this guidebook, we have commented extensively on the importance of preparation for any Everglades paddle trip—whether for a few hours or for several days. That information applies anytime, but there are some special considerations, additional equipment, and safety issues to factor in if you're setting out in the Everglades in June, July, or August.

WHY DO IT?

Why not? It's beautiful out there. Summer reveals still another of the many moods of the Everglades—bright and sparkling; colorful and changing; monumental clouds moving and sometimes issuing blue-black warnings; mangroves and islands awash in the summer abundance of water; marine mammals moving among bays; and herons and ibis, pelicans and shorebirds, ospreys and swallow-tailed kites dipping and diving. Compared with fall, winter, and spring, it's a quieter season on the water, even in the day-paddle areas, as there are fewer motorboats, and tour boats go out less often. You don't have to venture out as far to get the feeling of being in wilderness. While summer paddling in the Everglades should be undertaken thoughtfully, with careful planning and attention to safety, it can be fabulous.

THE HEAT

We generally don't feel the heat when we're on the water, especially in the vicinity of the Gulf or on Florida Bay, where there's almost always a breeze. But please follow the precautions we describe here.

▶ When you're on the water and there's a good breeze, you'll feel great, but this makes it all the more important to monitor your exposure time. The rays out there are intense, and you must be diligent about sun protection. Use sunscreen and lip balm with both UVA and UVB protection, and reapply the sunscreen and balm at least every 2 hours.

▶ Shade your face with a ventilated hat or a visor. Wear polarized sunglasses to protect your eyes.

▶ Ideally, wear lightweight long pants and a long-sleeved shirt, both of which are available permeated with sunscreen and insect repellent.

WATER, WATER, WATER!

The importance of staying hydrated cannot be overstated. Water is best, but you also may want to carry some electrolyte beverages (Gatorade, for example). Drink before you're thirsty. Repeat: Drink *before* you're thirsty. Try to drink at least every 15 minutes.

The standard guideline for a water supply is 1 gallon of water per person per day. In summer, that's not enough. You will need more water, especially if you're planning an overnight excursion and intend to make coffee or tea, or if you will use water in cooking. In those cases, take at least 1.5 gallons per person per day. It doesn't hurt to have more water than you think you'll need. Water makes great ballast.

COOLING STRATEGIES

Try the bandanna technique. Wet a bandanna and lay it on top of your head, under your hat or visor. Or wet it and tie it around your neck. You could also use two bandannas and do both.

Where you know it's safe—no motorboats in the way or alligators around—you may want to take a swim at some point in your paddle. If you don't want to take a swimsuit, just give yourself a good dunking in your clothes; they will dry quickly. Or you can just splash water on your clothes from time to time.

STRATEGIC FOOD PLANNING

Keep snacks handy in your craft. Water-rich fruits (such as apples and pre-peeled oranges) and protein-rich nuts are hydrating and nutritious choices. Snack often.

For dinner, keep it simple in summer, even if you're inclined to be an outdoor gourmet. After exerting yourself in heat during the day's paddle (although you may not feel it till you land), you might not be inclined to chop onions or prepare multiple dishes. Think about energy conservation (your own energy, that is).

INSECTS

They're out there, for sure. But with a few clever strategies and some special equipment, they become a manageable issue.

You are likely to have to deal with two kinds of insects: no-see-ums and mosquitoes. The no-see-ums are those tiny biting sand flies (also called midges) that you can't even see to swat, and, well, you know about mosquitoes (see page 254). In some areas, you may also encounter biting flies (see page 262).

You probably shouldn't try an overnight trip in summer if you can't stand being bitten at all by such insects, which live in the mangroves and on the islands. Mosquitoes and no-see-ums come out about the time the sun goes down and can be there in swarms until after the sun comes up. Even with all the strategies we recommend below, you're bound to get bitten a little (though perhaps no more than in a lot of backyards).

As for day paddles, these should be carefully selected because some paddles may take you into territory where the insects are out all day; others won't. Head toward open water for insect-free paddling during the day.

Repellents & Bites

This goes without saying, perhaps, but we'll say it anyway. Take insect repellent. Although many guides insist that only a repellent with DEET will work under Everglades-type conditions, recent research reports have found that other active ingredients, including lemon eucalyptus oil (now commercially available), are as effective as DEET, though for shorter periods of time. Combination sunscreen and insect repellent, with and without DEET, is available from several makers.

Regardless of any "foolproof" repellent, do carry anti-itch medications, such as Benadryl cream or its equivalent. It's inevitable that you will get a few bites, and you'll be glad you have some relief on hand.

Meshing It

A bug suit is essentially a fine-mesh net garment that you wear over your clothes to keep the insects out. You can purchase a whole suit or buy pieces separately—a head net, a bug jacket, and bug pants. You can even get bug socks. These should fit loosely, kind of balloon-like, over your clothes. If the mesh lies close to the skin, insects can still do their work on you. For summertime camping in the areas we describe, bug suits are a great source of comfort.

When planning for a summertime camping experience in the Everglades, be sure that the mesh of your tent screen is small enough to exclude no-see-ums. Not all tents are created equal in this regard.

Outwit the Bugs

If you have good insect repellent, a bug suit, a no-see-um-proof tent mesh, and a supply of Benadryl, you've done a lot to assure your comfort in the insect season. But you can take that even further:

First, for an overnight trip, time your paddle so that you don't end up cooking after dark—and plan to be comfortably inside your tent before dark. Try to reach your chickee or campsite early enough to cook dinner and clean up before the swarms arrive looking for their own dinner (that is, you). And be aware

Making coffee in bug suit

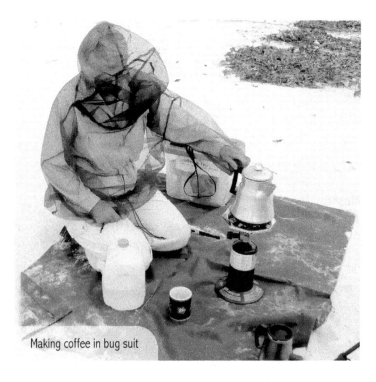

that mosquitoes prefer shade. If you pitch your tent in the shadiest spot, you are positioning yourself in the insects' favorite place.

The most challenging time for dealing with insects is overnight. If you're someone who never has to get up at night, then you are the perfect candidate for summer camping in the Everglades and environs. If you do have to step out of your tent before dawn, then put on your bug suit.

If you are a coffee drinker, you probably want coffee when the sun comes up. And often the mosquitoes don't want to go to bed by the time you want to get up. Sometimes a hopeful congregation of them will stay attached to the tent mesh well beyond the time when you want coffee. It actually works pretty well to put on the bug suit and go out to make coffee, but we've found another solution: a 24-hour thermos. Make coffee the night before, put it into the 24-hour thermos, and it's still steaming in the morning. Have early-morning coffee in the tent while the disappointed mosquitoes drift away to their daytime roosts. Then step outside and enjoy your bug-free day.

SUMMER ROUTES

In summer, the choice of route can matter in ways that transcend scenery. When deciding where you'll paddle, keep in mind conditions related to heat, insects, weather, and tide. If you want to paddle the entire 99-mile Wilderness Waterway in summer, careful planning is of urgent concern. When you're 5 days out and a yellow biting fly gets your ankles burning, there's no place to get the Benadryl you forgot to bring. If you didn't bring enough freshwater, the consequences can be deeply serious. Check, double-check, and triple-check your supplies before you head out, to be sure they can accommodate the period of time you expect your route to take. On the next page are two more guidelines for summer routing.

Choose Shorter Trips

In summer, most people will opt for shorter trips, which give less exposure to intense summer sun, greater comfort in relation to insects, and a better chance of paddling without having to deal with lightning. Further, we highly recommend that you plan for paddling *with* the tide, rather than against it. In summer, you want to be especially savvy about not exerting unnecessary effort beneath intense sun. Reducing your paddling time leads to a timely arrival at your destination, too, so you can have some fun exploring on land, fixing dinner, cleaning up, and getting inside the tent before the insects come.

Follow the Open Sky

You may want to make your short trips in the direction of the Gulf (when launching from Everglades City) or Florida Bay (when launching from Flamingo). On the rivers and in the backcountry, in dense mangrove areas not open to sun, the insects never seem to sleep. In those places, if you choose to go, you may need to wear your bug suit during the day. Toward the Gulf, however, or in Florida Bay, where there is plenty of moving air and open sky, you will generally encounter few or no insects while paddling.

SUMMER WEATHER

In any season for paddling in the Everglades, you will want to follow the weather reports and get to know the seasonal weather patterns. In summer, this is more important than ever. It is, after all, the rainy season, and rain clouds often deliver more than rain.

Lightning is a real threat that must not be taken lightly. We find that it is the most serious consideration of all. Be aware that the typical tropical summer weather pattern is a sunny morning with thunderstorms in the afternoon. With that in mind, an early launch is wise. Be aware, also, that there can be significant variations in this pattern. And if it's clear that there will be thunderstorms all day, or if the forecast indicates a high possibility of thunderstorms, the safe, wise thing to do is to *stay off the water.*

There are many summer days, however, when chances of scattered thundershowers are low or when there is no predicted storm activity at all. These can be great paddling days. With that in mind, we recommend the following precautions for dealing with the exigencies of summer weather.

Be a Radio Ranger

Before launching in the north or south Everglades, check forecasts at the Gulf Coast Visitor Center in Everglades City; at the Ernest F. Coe Visitor Center at the park entrance near Homestead; or at the Flamingo Visitor Center in Flamingo. Regardless of the forecast, carry a weather radio and use it. Short-term forecasts that detail the position and movement of thunderstorms are updated every hour. Know what's likely to be coming up within the next 24 hours, and keep in mind that conditions can change rapidly.

Be a Cloud Watcher

Stay alert for signs of imminent change. Make it a habit to check the sky in all directions—often. If you see thick, dark clouds forming in any direction, monitor them closely. If it becomes clear that they are moving in your direction (the weather radio can help you determine this), decide where you will head and what you will do if you begin to hear thunder.

Be a Lightning Mathematician

Thunder travels 1 mile every 5 seconds. If you see lightning, count the number of seconds before you hear thunder. Divide the number of seconds by 5, and you'll know the number of miles the lightning is from you. In quiet areas, like the ones in which you will be paddling, thunder can be heard for 10 miles. So if you counted 50 seconds, and divided it by 5, you would know that lightning is 10 miles away. Also, lightning can strike up to 10 miles from the area where it is raining. So if you're counting 50 or fewer seconds between lightning and thunder, you should carry out your lightning safety plan immediately.

There used to be a 30/30 rule—meaning that you would activate your safety plan at 30 seconds between lightning and thunder, and then take shelter until 30 minutes after the last bang. However, Jonathan Rizzo of the National Weather Service in Key West has advised us that the National Oceanic and Atmospheric Administration (NOAA) "has recently abandoned the full 30/30 rule, based on advice from William Roeder of the 45th Weather Squadron, a recognized lightning expert."

Instead, you should adopt the 50/30 rule: Take shelter if the flash-bang interval is 50 seconds or less. Remain in your protective position until 30 minutes after the last bang. Lightning can and often does strike within 30 minutes after the storm seems to have left. In short, Rizzo says, "NOAA has adopted [the guideline]: 'When thunder roars, go indoors.' The advice is [that] if you can hear thunder, you are close enough to be struck by lightning. So that's the point to begin seeking safe shelter."

Be a Squatter

During our first few years paddling in south Florida, mostly in the dry season, we often wondered aloud what we would do if we were caught in a thunderstorm. On land, we consulted books and asked a lot of people, "What do you do if you're out there and a thunderstorm comes up?"

The most frequent advice: "Get off the water immediately." But there is no land in some areas, only those impenetrable interlacings of mangrove prop roots known as mangrove islands. Getting off the water is not exactly an option. In that case, the advice is to get off the *expanse* of water: get to an edge and tuck the boat into an area of low mangroves, avoiding any individual tree that is higher than the others. Then keep yourself and your gear low in the boat and wait until the storm has completely blown over.

If you are on land or can get to land before the storm strikes, avoid the open beach or other exposed area. Seek low vegetation and minimize your contact with the earth. This translates into what is known as the lightning crouch: squat, tuck, and cover.

- *Squat* on the ground, keeping your feet close together. If you have a sleep mat handy, you can squat on the mat.
- *Tuck* your head down.
- *Cover* your ears with your hands and open your mouth for protection from changes in air pressure.

The lightning crouch advice replaces the old maxim of lying flat on the ground, an act that gets you low but increases your exposure to ground currents. And it definitely supersedes heading for the cone of protection you may have heard about—an area within 45 degrees of a tall, isolated object in which lighting will not strike. That one is a myth.

One more note: If you are with companions, do not cluster together during the storm (though that might be your impulse). Spread out. You will be less likely to attract a strike separately than you will together.

Be a Responsible Companion

Before you head out, discuss with your paddling companion(s) what you will do if you have to deal with lightning during your adventure. As you paddle, communicate about what you observe in the clouds. When you set up camp, talk about what you will do if a storm comes up in the night. Don't wait to confront it until you are within the 50/30 zone or until you wake up in the night with thunder crashing around you. (In the latter case, keep in mind that a tent offers no protection.)

Get CPR training and keep it up to date. With CPR administered quickly, very few people die of lightning strike. And don't worry about getting a shock from the body of a person who has been struck. It won't happen. As stated on the FEMA website **fema.gov/hazard/thunderstorm**, "Lightning strike victims carry no electrical charge and should be tended to immediately."

Lightning Watchword

These notes on lightning may be sobering. They should be. Lightning is dangerous. Be informed, be aware, and be careful. We haven't let the high frequency of storms in Florida's summers keep us from paddling, but we are hyperalert in summer. And when we *know* a storm is out there, we don't go.

Part Five:

The Campsites

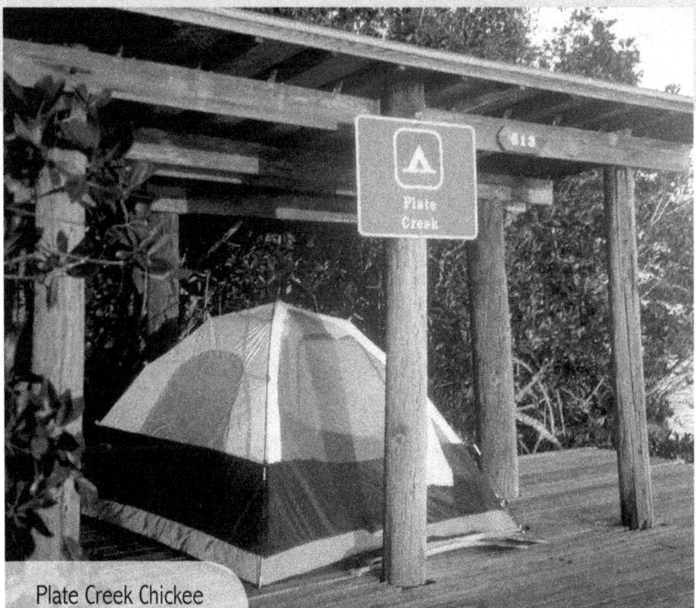

Plate Creek Chickee

The following are descriptions of National Park Service (NPS) campsites referred to in this book. They are listed in alphabetical order with corresponding map locators for reader convenience. Wherever "privy" is noted, there is only one. *Remember that you must make reservations at the Gulf Coast Visitor Center or the Flamingo Visitor Center within 24 hours of the trip during which you plan to use these sites.*

ALLIGATOR CREEK (ground site)

Map Locator: Overnight Paddles, West Lake to Alligator Creek (page 197)
Maximum number of people: 8
Maximum number of parties: 3
Maximum number of nights: 2
Facilities: No dock, privy, or picnic tables

▶ Located where Alligator Creek meets Garfield Bight, this campsite sits on a marl prairie covered with sea purslane and glasswort, dotted by black mangroves.

Take care when you step out of your boat and onto the marl at your landing here. Marl is a gray, limy mud that is formed when calcite crystals mix with the algae formation called periphyton. When wet, marl is slippery. In *A Dredgeman of Cape Sable,* a reminiscence of his 1922 work on a floating dredge in the Glades, author Lawrence E. Will said of marl, "When dry it made a right good road, but when wet—oh, brother—greased glass couldn't be any slicker!"

Alligator Creek Campsite has an open feel with its views across the expanse of green ground cover, but camping here can be buggy. This is a good spot for a bug suit.

Because of the shallow waters of Garfield Bight, motorboaters usually don't venture to this campsite, so it is one of the lesser-used sites in the park. If you do have company, expect close quarters, as the campsite is quite small.

Bring your binoculars to do some birding, either by paddling a bit into the bight if the tide is up or walking down one of the paths that lead to the black mangroves along the bight. There you can catch glimpses of roseate spoonbills (see page 259), stilts, white pelicans in season, and a great variety of other wading birds and shorebirds. Although you do not have an unobstructed view of the birds on Garfield Bight from the campsite itself, you will have a narrow but nonetheless spectacular view of the sunset.

Holly's journal entry: *What noise last night—birds flapping to roost, barred owls calling to one another, fish splashing in the creek, mosquitoes whining. I'm amazed I slept at all.*

Tent in sea purslane prairie at Alligator Creek

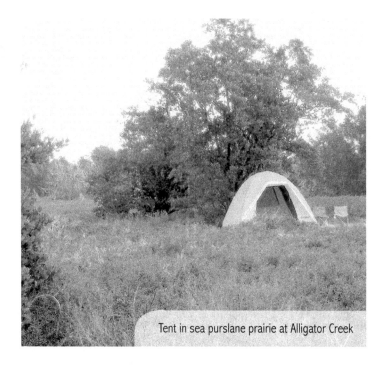

BROAD RIVER (ground site)

Map Locator: Sections 12/J (page 91), 13/I (page 92), & 14/H (page 95)
Maximum number of people: 10
Maximum number of parties: 3
Maximum number of nights: 2
Facilities: Dock with slanted ramp, privy, & 2 picnic tables

▶ For many traveling north to south, the Broad River Campsite is the staging area for paddling The Nightmare. The campsite is located just east of marker 25, which signals the entrance to Wood River, where The Nightmare begins.

If you are traveling south to north, this campsite might be your resting place after a day of paddling Broad Creek and The Nightmare.

Because the Broad River Campsite is close to the Gulf of Mexico, the L-shaped dock has a slanted ramp, built to accommodate loading and unloading your gear in this area of great tidal fluctuation. Navigating the dock onto the campsite is tricky, so use caution.

Anne's journal entry: *When we were on the dock and it was getting dark, Holly heard them before I saw them—ibis flying up the river, low over the water's surface, hundreds, then thousands of them coming and coming, and then some of them began to settle into trees on the opposite bank. We sat in silence and watched.*

CAMP LONESOME (ground site)

Map Locator: Section 12/J (page 91)
Maximum number of people: 10
Maximum number of parties: 3
Maximum number of nights: 3
Facilities: Dock, privy, & 2 picnic tables

▶ Camp Lonesome, located on a Calusa (see page 247) shell mound, is set back in the mangrove shoreline. From a small dock, the pier leads to a shaded area with two alcoves—one left, one right, with two picnic tables in the middle. The left-alcove vegetation includes the red-barked gumbo limbo (see page 251) and spreading mahogany trees, as well as the oval-leaved pigeon plum that produces a berrylike fruit that pigeons love to eat. On the right, hear the rustle of cabbage palms (Florida's state tree) and smell the earthy scent of white stoppers. Look carefully everywhere for a fringe of poison ivy.

Holly's journal entry: *We ate dinner on the dock, watching flocks of swallows dart overhead catching insects.*

CANEPATCH (ground site)

Map Locator: Sections 15/G (page 99) & 16/F (page 101)
Maximum number of people: 12
Maximum number of parties: 4
Maximum number of nights: 3
Facilities: Dock with multiple boat cleats, privy, & 2 picnic tables

▶ Here you will enjoy close contact with the interior of the Everglades. The small lagoon in front of the dock may be busy with birds and fish. The water is quite fresh here. We have seen alligators here and, once, a large dolphin fishing vigorously for a couple of hours before dark.

Scattered sugarcane plants, as well as banana, guava, lime, and avocado trees, mingle among native species on this site, which has known a variety of agricultural uses by both Native Americans and white settlers. You may also spot nickerbean plants (see page 255), sprawling with their spiny seedpods. Be alert for poison ivy.

Holly's journal entry: *A lighted jet just flew overhead, and I am thinking of those passengers disembarking in the glare and bustle of Miami, while here we are, tucked quietly into a tent at Canepatch deep in the Everglades.*

CROOKED CREEK CHICKEE (double platform)

Map Locator: Sections 2/T (page 62) & 3/S (page 64); Overnight Paddles, Hurddles Creek Loop (page 141)
Maximum number of people: 6 on each platform
Maximum number of parties: 2
Maximum number of nights: 1
Facilities: Dock (with ladder) & privy

▶ Nestled behind a mangrove island, away from the main flow of the Lopez River, Crooked Creek Chickee offers a tranquil retreat in the mangroves.

Crooked Creek Chickee was constructed in 2011 to replace Sunday Bay Chickee, which had long been a favorite first-night stop for southbound paddlers. Over time the shallow waters in front of Sunday Bay Chickee silted up and the chickee itself was often inaccessible. The water is shallow at Crooked Creek Chickee, too, but you won't have to worry about getting stuck at low tide, and you'll spend the night just a small island away from an important, historic artery connecting the Gulf region with the interior. This chickee is quite accessible for an overnight trip from Chokoloskee. It's an easy first-night stop if you're heading south on the Waterway or a

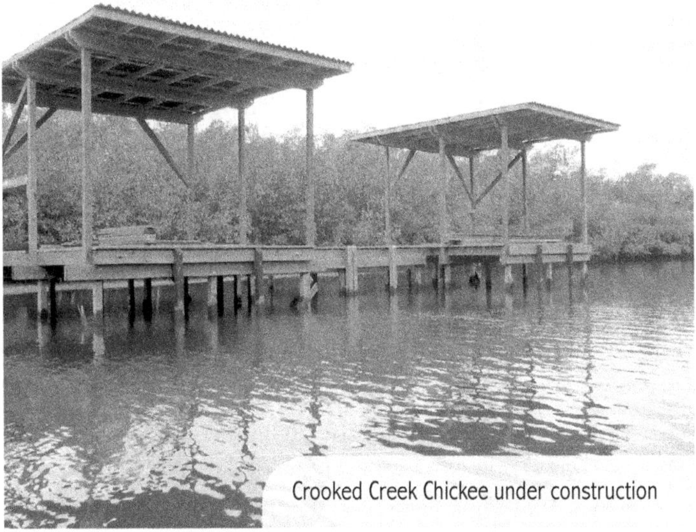

Crooked Creek Chickee under construction

good place to pause before making the transition to the "ordinary world" after a thru-paddle from Flamingo.

DARWIN'S PLACE (ground site)

Map Locator: Sections 5/Q (page 69) & 6/P (page 73)
Maximum number of people: 8
Maximum number of parties: 2
Maximum number of nights: 3
Facilities: Dock, privy, & 3 picnic tables

▶ Just past marker 97 and directly on the Waterway, Darwin's Place on Opossum Key is a Calusa shell mound homesteaded by mid-20th-century settlers, such as Arthur Darwin, for whom it is named.

In the late 1800s, plumer Jean Chevelier lived on Opossum Key and later, in the early 1930s, Glades memoirist Totch Brown and his family stayed on the site for a while. As he wrote in his 1993 book, *Totch: A Life in the Everglades*, "It's a good piece of high land, and one of the flatter-type mounds. The Indians who built it really knew their stuff. They picked out a nice harbor pass, plenty deep at any stage of tide, out of the north wind and good for the summer breeze, and not far to go for fresh water."

Today, you can see the tabby foundation (see page 262) for the homesite of Darwin, who claimed to be a fifth-generation descendent of the geneticist Charles Darwin. Living on this island from 1945 to his death in 1977 at the reported age of 112, Arthur Darwin grew vegetables and bananas and raised rabbits. He lived in a concrete blockhouse with no running water or electricity, gathered rainwater in his cistern, and reportedly killed great numbers of opossums. The pamphlet "Hermits from the Mangrove Country of the Everglades" reports on Darwin's 1980 interview with Everglades City High School students, during which he acknowledged that he came to the island not to "get away from the world. I just like it here." (Visit **hermitary.com.**)

Today, the place that Darwin "just liked" is overgrown with vegetation, making it quite buggy. One late April, we were bothered by yellow flies (see page 262) when we stopped for lunch, and we moved on in a hurry.

Holly's journal entry: *Anne and I have been poking around the tabby remains on Darwin's old homestead. It's hard to imagine this overgrown area opened up enough to farm.*

HARNEY RIVER CHICKEE (double platform)

Map Locator: Sections 14/H (page 95) & 15/G (page 99)
Maximum number of people: 6 on each platform
Maximum number of parties: 2
Maximum number of nights: 1
Facilities: Dock (with ladder) & privy

▶ With marker 12 nailed to its side, the Harney River Chickee lies at the spot where Broad Creek empties into the Harney River. North-to-south paddlers will relax on this reconstructed chickee after having paddled The Nightmare and Broad Creek. South-to-north paddlers will use this as the staging spot before tackling these two twisting waterways.

The tidal fluctuation at this chickee is great. When you land you might wonder at the reason for the sturdy ladders, but you will see the need when you try to load your boat in the

Home sweet home on Harney River Chickee

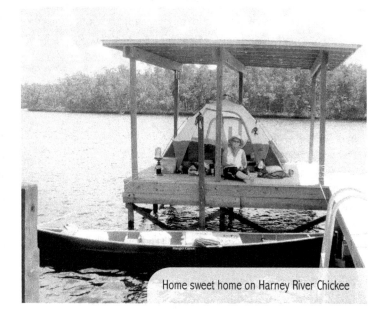

morning. This is one site where you must leave sufficient slack in your tie ropes and watch that your boat does not get wedged under the chickee boards or isn't left hanging in the air on too-short ropes.

Out in the Harney River, across from the chickee, is an ibis roost (see page 252). The numbers of ibis coming and going from this island will vary. We have seen dozens of them and, on one dramatic occasion, thousands of them. Watching flocks land in the trees in the evening and take off to feed in the morning offers some of the best of Everglades entertainment.

This chickee was originally a single and located on Ibis Island. On older maps, you may see it positioned there. It had become unstable and was rebuilt off the direct flow of the Harney at this more sheltered spot. Fortunately the new chickee is a double because this site is in high demand.

Anne's journal entry: *Dirt daubers seem to love these chickees. The underside of the roof of this one is covered with their mud constructions. Occasionally we see one of the busy daubers, but they haven't bothered us.*

HELLS BAY CHICKEE (double platform)

Map Locator: Overnight Paddles, Hells Bay Canoe Trail (page 179)
Maximum number of people: 6 on each platform
Maximum number of parties: 2
Maximum number of nights: 1
Facilities: Dock & privy

▶ Hells Bay Chickee lies at the end of the marked Hells Bay Canoe Trail. It is a popular stopping place for motorboaters coming from Whitewater Bay and for paddlers reaching the end of the marked canoe trail, so you will likely have company.

You can see the fishermen's influence, with a PVC fishing-pole holder and a mercury-level warning sign on the right (north) chickee. These chickee platforms face east, away from the shoreline; this location, coupled with a breeze, may make for fewer mosquitoes. On a clear night you will see innumerable stars and a glow in the east from Miami, and in the morning you will wake up to sunrise in front of your tent.

Holly's journal entry: *Out on the bay there is a luminous reflection of clouds and sky in the rippling water.*

HIGHLAND BEACH (beach site)

Map Locator: Section 13/I (page 92)
Maximum number of people: 24
Maximum number of parties: 4
Maximum number of nights: 3
Facilities: No dock, privy, or picnic tables

▶ When you have found a place along the beach that you would like to adopt as your site, tie up to a palm tree or a heavy piece of driftwood or flotsam that is embedded in the sand; you can sense the high-tide line by the edge of dry debris, the wrack line. Then watch the tides so you don't have to drag your boat out into the water when you are ready to launch.

Highland Beach is one of our favorite campsites. Sunsets on the Gulf are amazing, and here we have witnessed the green flash, that ephemeral spectacle of light at sunset or sunrise. Once, while preparing dinner at Highland Beach, we watched a doe and two fawns coming down to the water's edge.

Early Calusa and pioneer hunters, explorers, and fishermen traveled this beach, which stretches south from Lostmans River to the Broad River. When settlers Wallace Rewis and his wife farmed here during the 1930s, it was called Lostmans Beach. At one time there were stately royal palms on the ridge behind the beachfront, but these have disappeared, some carried off to line the streets of Fort Myers, Florida, in an earlier age.

Like all beaches, Highland changes over time and in response to storms. It has changed significantly just in the years we've been paddling there. Dramatic storm erosion has left the root masses of some cabbage palms exposed, making it difficult for us to locate sites where we had previously camped.

Vegetation here is, of course, a different mix from the interior sites and includes seaside purslane, Spanish bayonet, coral bean, seashore saltgrass, railroad vine, and sida, along with familiar cabbage palms. And watch out for sand spurs. If you enjoy shelling, this is a great place, but remember not to take live shells.

Launching in the morning will be either tricky or simple, depending on the tides and the weather. We have launched from Highland Beach when the Gulf was as smooth as sea glass, and there have also been times when we had to be careful because of the waves.

If you are paddling north to south, be sure to time your departure from Highland Beach according to the tides, assuring that you will not be stuck in The Nightmare at low tide.

Anne's journal entry: *The osprey hovers, makes a dart of himself, splashes, disappears momentarily—then floats, flaps his wings and lifts, laboring a little with the heavy load in his talons, then gives a shake and flies away.*

JEWELL KEY (beach site)

Map Locator: Overnight Paddles, Jewell Key (page 150)
Maximum number of people: 8
Maximum number of parties: 2
Maximum number of nights: 2
Facilities: Privy

▶ Jewell Key is one of the newest campsites in the park, replacing the chickee at Kingston Key that Hurricane Wilma destroyed. The campsite lies at the northern end of the island, and from your site you will watch sunrise rather than sunset because the camping area faces the mainland, not the Gulf. Camping is not permitted on the Gulf side, so set up your tent on the small beach or tucked up near the mangroves.

A stay at Jewell Key offers multiple enchantments: birdwatching, beachcombing, fishing in the cove by the campsite or out in the Gulf, or relaxing with a book on the beach. Spend some time examining the vegetation. Mangroves anchor the island, and the Gulf side offers seagrapes and twists of buttonwoods.

The patch of growth between the privy and the tide line provides a ragged garden of some of the most salt-tolerant, beach-binding plants in the ecosystem. It includes railroad vine, which sends out long runners to hold down the sand, sometimes offering lavender blooms. Sea purslane—with its narrow, fleshy leaves and diminutive flowers—also helps to anchor the beach, sprawling and sending down roots from the nodes. Seashore salt grass works underground, forming thick entanglements of rhizomes. Coast spurge gets into the act, looking herblike, but don't even think about tasting it. Its leaves, seeds, and milky white sap are toxic. Look closely, and you'll see a few tufts of blue porterweed, along with some wild sage.

While Jewell Key is a lovely spot to camp, be sure to pull your boat up out of the reach of the tides and secure your food and water from the rats that inhabit this island.

Anne's journal entry: *We made rooibos tea and sat in front of the tent watching a father and small son fish, watching the pelicans dive, watching a dark cloud in the northwest.*

Holly's journal entry: *Picking my way through mudflat and worm rock, I walked this morning around the edge of the key to the Gulf of Mexico. The tide was low, exposing whelk and oyster shells, and the twisted shapes of buttonwood.*

JOE RIVER CHICKEE (double platform)

Map Locator: Sections 18/D (page 107) & 19/C (page 109)
Maximum number of people: 6 on each platform
Maximum number of parties: 2
Maximum number of nights: 1
Facilities: Dock (with ladder) & privy

▶ Unlike many of the chickees, this one is clearly visible from the main channel, the Joe River. A convenient feature is the shelves built on each of the chickee platforms. This is a pretty spot for exploration, with small channels opening in the mangroves around it.

Although we have never had trouble with insects here, we've heard reports of this site being buggier than most chickees. One blogger wrote of a January visit, "As we approached the chickee platform the mob of no-see-ums descended upon us."

Anne's journal entry: *I've been lying stomach down on the boards for nearly an hour, listening to the wind, that tone, which I know I will long for when I am gone. Between the boards, through wide cracks, I watch the water dappling.*

Holly's journal entry: *As we paddled up, three dolphins, two large and one small, raced past us out of the creek to the northwest side of the chickee. One tilted its head and looked at us with one large eye.*

JOHNSON KEY CHICKEE (double platform)

Map Locator: Overnight Paddles, Johnson Key (page 184)
Maximum number of people: 6 on each platform
Maximum number of parties: 2
Maximum number of nights: 1
Facilities: Boat slips, aluminum ladders, wooden slat ladders, railings, ropes to hoist gear, a dock, & privy

▶ It's an effort to get up here, but the view from this chickee makes it all worthwhile. To the north you will see the end of mainland Florida, to the east Johnson Key, to the south Man of War Key, and all around you the expanse of Florida Bay. Below you lie lush seagrass meadows (see page 259) waving in the current that flows through the clear, shallow waters of the bay.

It is because of the seagrass that this chickee stands so high and the boards are spaced so far apart. Regulations require that the platforms be elevated 5 or more feet above the water and that boards be spaced wide so that sunlight can reach the grass.

Aluminum ladders extend from the boat slips to the chickee platforms, and ropes are attached to the chickee to help lift your gear to the decks. NPS has added a dock with aluminum ladders to make things even easier. Wooden 2-by-4-foot slats form ladders on the south side of the platforms. Pack light to ease the chore of lifting supplies onto the chickee platforms.

The posts and boards by the boat slips are encrusted with barnacles, so we suggest bringing boat bumpers or milk jugs to serve as bumpers to prevent scratches on the sides of your craft.

Also bring a cooking tarp to spread out so that your utensils don't drop between the chickee boards. At times there has

Dan and Casey at Johnson Key

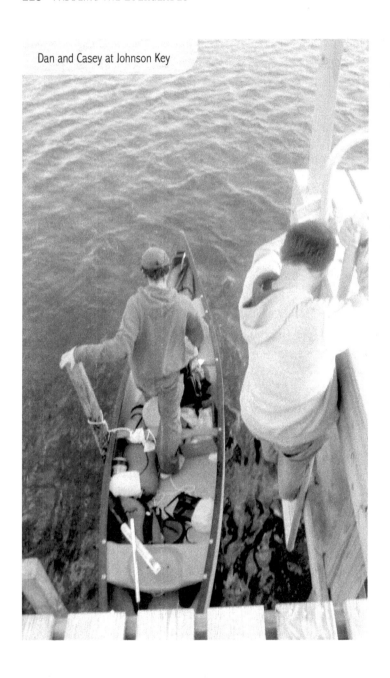

been a concern about excessive bird droppings, as this campsite provides a perfect perch for pelicans. A tarp will be a help if the platforms are messy.

Because your tent is sitting high over Florida Bay and you might be camping in strong winds, consider anchoring the corners of your tent to the uprights with ropes or bungee cords. But the winds are a blessing because mosquitoes won't be a problem at Johnson Key.

Holly's journal entry: *How beautiful this is—the water flowing beneath this tall chickee, the sky reddening as the sun begins to set. I feel as if I'm going to sleep on a ship out in Florida Bay tonight.*

LARD CAN (ground site)

Map Locator: Overnight Paddles, Hells Bay Canoe Trail (page 179)
Maximum number of people: 10
Maximum number of parties: 4
Maximum number of nights: 2
Facilities: Dock & privy

▶ In her 1947 classic, *The Everglades: River of Grass,* Marjory Stoneman Douglas explains that the word *hammock* comes from the Arawak word *hamaca,* meaning "jungle or masses of vegetation floating in a tropical river." Set on a tropical hardwood hammock (see page 251), Lard Can is often muddy and can be completely flooded and closed after heavy rains. In the summertime, mosquitoes will be a problem here. But for many there is a certain pleasure, a sense of historical and emotional connection, that comes from camping where Native Americans and pioneers have spent time.

When you arrive, pull up to the dock by the open tenting area; a second, drier tent site lies to the right, and the privy is to the left. Whether you camp or simply explore Lard Can, take note of the variety of plants that inhabit this higher ground—cocoplum, sawgrass, cabbage palms, and ferns.

Holly's journal entry: *This land has a tale to tell, the stories of all the people who have stayed here, from the Calusa to the pioneers to the present-day paddlers. The people are here and then disappear, but the mangrove and buttonwood and sabal palm remain.*

LOPEZ RIVER (ground site)

Map Locator: Sections 2/T (page 62) & 3/S (page 64); Day Paddles, Lopez River Route (page 127); Overnight Paddles, Hurddles Creek (page 141)
Maximum number of people: 12
Maximum number of parties: 3
Maximum number of nights: 2
Facilities: Privy & 2 picnic tables

▶ Approximately 8 miles from Everglades City, the Lopez River Campsite marks the homestead of Gregorio Lopez. Arriving from Spain in the 1890s, Lopez settled on this Calusa shell mound along the river that today bears his name. He was an early Everglades plumer, a man who hunted American egrets, snowy egrets, and sometimes pink roseate spoonbills to harvest plumes for ladies' hats—a fashion rage in those days.

To catch rainwater, as freshwater was scarce in this region, Lopez built the large cistern that you still see today. Settlers on other islands, as well as hunters in the area, sometimes came here for water. You will also see two concrete vaults in front of the cistern, one marked with an inscription that, in part, reads "Lopes [sic] Born April 29, 1892."

The old concrete cistern and an NPS sign make the campsite easy to spot at the side of the river. As with most of the ground sites on the Waterway, you'll land your boat on a hard-packed shell beach. However, in the rainy season (summer) the campsite itself can be quite muddy.

Holly's journal entry: *This is not an isolated place; powerboats are passing regularly. I think this must have been a busy spot in Lopez's day too, with Chokoloskee and Everglades City nearby. An easier spot to live, I'm thinking, than at Canepatch or Camp Lonesome.*

LOSTMANS FIVE (ground site)

Map Locator: Sections 7/O (page 76) & 8/N (page 79)
Maximum number of people: 10
Maximum number of parties: 2
Maximum number of nights: 3
Facilities: Dock, 2 tent platforms, privy, 2 picnic tables

▶ Lostmans Five Campsite sits on the shore of Lostmans Five Bay and at the mouth of Lostmans Five River. At the water's edge, you'll see the broken concrete remains from early land-speculation offices that once sat on this site.

Charlton Tebeau, in his *Man in the Everglades,* relates two of the possible explanations for the name Lostmans. One suggestion is that the river was named for a Seminole War Army surgeon, Thomas Lawson, with the name changing over time to Lostman; another is that Lostmans was named for five Army deserters escaping from Key West who were put off at the side of the river and told that they might find work at a sawmill back in the woods.

There are perks to staying at Lostmans Five. It is nice to have such easy access to your boat, and the sunsets from the Lostmans Five dock are spectacular.

Holly's journal entry: *The Milky Way is spread over the Everglades tonight.*

OYSTER BAY CHICKEE (double platform)

Map Locator: Sections 17/E (page 104) & 18/D (page 107)
Maximum number of people: 6 on each platform
Maximum number of parties: 2
Maximum number of nights: 1
Facilities: Dock (with ladder) & privy

▶ Look for this chickee inside a cluster of islands about 0.5 mile southwest of U.S. Coast Guard (USCG) marker 50. The site can be a bit tricky to find, so please carefully read the paddling directions on pages 103–108 for this area of the Wilderness Waterway.

The chickee has a nice, sheltered feel to it. It would seem that fish like this area, too, because fishers of all kinds show up here—brown pelicans, kingfishers, anhingas, great blue herons, dolphins, and, occasionally, humans. The more northern of the two platforms has a shelf, convenient for stand-up cooking, as opposed to kneeling by your campstove.

Anne's journal entry: *Fish jump all around us—small splashes. The sky is thick with stars. Those fish sounds are interesting—more than the simple sound of a fish lifting out of the water, then reentering. It's almost as though the fish gives itself a shake while out of water.*

PEARL BAY CHICKEE (double platform)

Map Locator: Overnight Paddles, Hells Bay Canoe Trail (page 179)
Maximum number of people: 6 on each platform
Maximum number of parties: 2
Maximum number of nights: 1
Facilities: Boat slip, large platforms, & large privy, all handicap accessible with guardrails or handrails

▶ Pearl Bay is the largest of the park's chickees and the only one that is handicap-accessible. This double chickee has wooden guardrails most of the way around and a covered boat slip with aluminum handrails and steps, making for easy access to your canoe or kayak. The privy is a large wooden structure, built to handle a wheelchair. The chickee faces south across the bay and backs up against a mangrove island.

In *Words on the Wilderness,* author Larry Perez suggests that the name Pearl Bay might refer to an area where Native Americans gathered pearl-bearing oysters. You may not spot oysters below the chickee these days, but you will see hydrilla, an invasive water plant brought in on boat propellers.

Holly's journal entry: *There is a sliver of a moon tonight and a spangle of stars over Pearl Bay Chickee.*

PICNIC KEY (beach site)

Map Locator: Overnight Paddles, Indian Key Pass (page 145)
Maximum number of people: 16
Maximum number of parties: 3
Maximum number of nights: 3
Facilities: Privy

▶ Backed by seagrapes, beach spider lilies, nickerbean (see page 255), inkberry, and mangrove, Picnic Key Campsite lies on a stretch of beach on the southwest side of the key. Memoirist Totch Brown recounted that this was a site of "sea-graping" in his youth. He wrote, "We'd spread a blanket under a grape tree, shake the tree, and then dump the fruit from the blanket into a washtub. Back home, the women cooked 'em up into sea-grape jelly, and was it ever good."

Set up your tent in one of the various clearings back in the vegetation area, or camp right on the beach, making sure to pitch your tent above the wrack line (that strip of dried vegetation left at high tide) so you don't wake up with wet feet. Although you cannot see the sunset from this campsite because Tiger Key lies to the west, you have a wide-open view of the Gulf, with its color variations under the changing sunlight and clouds.

If you land at low tide, be sure to pull up and tie your boat so you don't find it floating away when the tide comes in. Also, when you land or launch or wish to cool off with a swim, wear shoes to protect your feet from the jagged worm rock (see page 264).

When camping at Picnic Key, you might want to pack a little whisk broom and dustpan if sand in the tent bothers you: the sand is quartz, powder-fine, clingy, and almost impossible to keep out.

Anne's journal entry: *This island is bursting with seagrape. I've put my chair in the shade of a spreading tree, pressed in among the thick leaves and waterfalls of hard green grape.*

Holly's journal entry: *As I was beach walking this morning, I saw a broad track in the sand from the water to above the high-tide line. A sea turtle came in to lay her eggs while we were sleeping last night.*

PLATE CREEK CHICKEE (single platform)

Map Locator: Sections 7/O (page 76) & 8/N (page 79)
Maximum number of people: 6
Maximum number of parties: 1
Maximum number of nights: 1
Facilities: Dock & privy

▶ This single-platform chickee is unusually roomy. It has a side platform about 6 feet wide that extends beyond the roofed area of the chickee.

One of the oldest chickees in the park, Plate Creek was built on the remnants of the Poinciana Land Development Company. Staying here gives you a feel for that part of Everglades history. In fact, if you peek under the chickee, you'll see some of the original wooden posts. The NPS has added reinforced pilings, maintaining the chickee's history while keeping campers safe.

When planning to camp here, be sure to bring your kitchen tarp to keep things from falling through the wide gaps between the boards of this chickee.

Anne's journal entry: *Dolphins. We watched them swimming fast, pushing up water, then surfacing, blowing. This trip, there has been no day without dolphins. We have been dolphin rich.*

RODGERS RIVER CHICKEE (double platform)

Map Locator: Sections 10/L (page 84) & 11/K (page 87)
Maximum number of people: 6 on each platform
Maximum number of parties: 2
Maximum number of nights: 1
Facilities: Dock (with ladder) & privy

▶ Perched at an edge of a wide bay, Rodgers River Chickee sits in a windy spot. Often there is a visible current, and sometimes whitecaps, running through the bay. Each time we have stayed on this chickee, we have listened to our canoe bump through the night, no matter what side of the chickee we tied it to.

In addition, the chickee's roof has a crossbeam on which we were constantly banging our heads.

Despite the windy tendencies here, we have seen early mornings when the water was as smooth as silk. Here, we have known the company of dolphins and croaking herons, and in the evening, the music of insects and frogs. You are deep in wilderness at Rodgers River Chickee.

Anne's journal entry: *I know my smallness here, my frailty. I am in awe of the universe.*

SHARK POINT CHICKEE (double platform)

Map Locator: Overnight Paddles, Shark Point (page 188)
Maximum number of people: 6 on each platform
Maximum number of parties: 2
Maximum number of nights: 1
Facilities: Boat slips, aluminum ladders, wooden slat ladders, railings, ropes to hoist gear, dock, & privy

▶ One of the newest chickees in the park, Shark Point Chickee takes the place of the Shark Point Campsite. In order to provide necessary light to the seagrass beds, this chickee sits high, making it tricky to unload gear, and the boards are spaced an inch apart, so watch that your gear doesn't fall between the slats.

In spite of the inconvenience that high chickees with widely spaced boards can present, the perspective from the deck is excellent. You have fine views of both sunrise and sunset.

The wildlife viewing is equally enthralling here: watching the seagrass meadows (see page 259) is almost hypnotic as you keep looking to see what might pass by. If you're lucky, you may even spot small sharks at Shark Point Chickee.

The chickee is equipped with tall aluminum ladders on each platform as well as a deck with aluminum ladders. The NPS has added ropes to the chickees to help hoist your supplies.

Pelicans and cormorants use this chickee as a roost when you're not there, and you might spot pelicans floating nearby, annoyed by your invasion. You may also find bird droppings along the boardwalk to the privy, but probably not on your sleeping platform, which is covered by the chickee roof.

You will want to spread a tarp to keep smaller gear from falling through the spaces between the chickee boards. You might also bring along bumpers or plastic jugs to protect your boat from the barnacles on the pilings.

Anne's journal entry: *Bald eagle over Shark Point. A pair of ospreys shriek and give chase. One of them dives into the eagle midair. They recover from the collision, and pursuit resumes.*

Holly's journal entry: *If this amazing place hadn't been preserved as a national park, we would be seeing condos and high-rises and resorts lining the shores at Shark Point rather than watching a darkening shoreline and the stars coming out over Florida Bay tonight.*

SHARK RIVER CHICKEE (single platform)

Map Locator: Sections 16/F (page 101) & 17/E (page 104)
Maximum number of people: 6
Maximum number of parties: 1
Maximum number of nights: 1
Facilities: Dock (with ladder) & privy

▶ Built on a side channel off the Little Shark River, this chickee is one of the oldest in the park and is set close to the arching prop roots of the red mangroves (see page 253). Your ears and eyes will have an ideal vantage point as you listen for mangrove crabs scuttling around on the deck, spot a blue crab swimming below, or watch a group of ibis preening in puddles behind the chickee before flying off to roost.

Be aware, however, that this chickee is in shallow water. In winter, at low tide, it might be surrounded by mudbanks, making it difficult or impossible to land or embark without waiting for a tide change.

Holly's journal entry: *Six white ibis just marched through the mangroves behind the chickee. Honking and preening, they splash in a little pool they've found.*

SOUTH JOE RIVER CHICKEE (double platform)

Map Locator: Sections 19/C (page 109) & 20/B (page 112); Overnight Paddles, South Joe River (page 193)
Maximum number of people: 6 on each platform
Maximum number of parties: 2
Maximum number of nights: 1
Facilities: Dock (with ladder) & privy

▶ This is the closest chickee to Flamingo, about 10 miles away, and in some seasons it gets heavy use. It is somewhat exposed, due to its position toward the front of a large cove. There are often high winds here, especially in the afternoons. As a safeguard, we usually bungee all four corners of our tent to the chickee posts.

Sunrise is lovely here, and we have enjoyed watching dolphins play. Once, we were visited by a large sphinx moth. At various times of year we have heard the sounds of crow, woodpecker, and great horned owl. And, on occasion, our visitors have included mosquitoes, though the wind, when it is blowing, does keep them at bay.

Anne's journal entry: *Sunrise began as a long orange band over the mangroves. Now, a golden light spreads over everything.*

SWEETWATER CHICKEE (double platform)

Map Locator: Sections 5/Q (page 69) & 6/P (page 73)
Maximum number of people: 6 on each platform
Maximum number of parties: 2
Maximum number of nights: 1
Facilities: Dock (with ladder) & privy

▶ Hard to find, Sweetwater Chickee is worth the effort. It is in an isolated spot, located on Sweetwater Creek behind an island with palm trees. Memoirist Totch Brown, in his stories of boyhood days in the Everglades, talks of the Seminoles having named the narrow little river on which the chickee sits Sweetwater because it is more fresh than salty. He describes Sweetwater as running from the Glades down to the mangroves, and remembers that when he and his family stayed on Opossum Key, they would take their skiff to get freshwater from Sweetwater.

In spring we've had yellow flies here (see page 262) and have heard the buzz of mosquitoes outside our tent after dark. An odder sound was a hum like a generator, which we determined was the sound of frogs in the sawgrass that lies behind the mangroves. One time when we stayed on this chickee, we heard a rage of splashing during the evening, went out of our tent, and shined our headlamps onto the water. The eyes of alligators reflected red everywhere, alligators in a feeding frenzy, hunting in the water around and under our chickee. It was the only time we've ever witnessed that phenomenon. If you are fortunate enough to have an experience like this, put on your headlamp and enjoy it. The alligators are interested in fish, not you. And be comforted in knowing that in the morning, all will be calm and you will have a quiet paddle back down Sweetwater Creek.

Holly's journal entry: *We've been listening to fish jumping after insects tonight, making mad water music around the chickee.*

THE WATSON PLACE (ground site)

Map Locator: Sections 5/Q (page 69) & 6/P (page 73)
Maximum number of people: 20
Maximum number of parties: 5
Maximum number of nights: 2
Facilities: Dock, privy, & 3 picnic tables

▶ The story goes that The Watson Place is haunted. This campsite, 1.5 miles down the Chatham River from marker 100, sits on the old homestead of "Bloody Ed" Watson. Made famous in Peter Matthiessen's 1990 bestseller, *Killing Mister Watson*, the homesteader is said to have "done in" his laborers rather than pay them. Unquestionably the most notorious of the early Everglades pioneers, Watson was rumored to have killed the Oklahoma outlaw Belle Starr, as well as numerous others with whom he had altercations. Fed up with what they believed were his crimes, the residents took the law into their own hands and confronted him outside Smallwood Store on Chokoloskee on October 27, 1910, killing Watson in a barrage of bullets.

Watson's farm on Chatham Bend was prosperous and, at 35 acres, large by Everglades standards. He grew vegetables and produced a fine sugarcane syrup called Island Pride. You can

Campers at Sweetwater Chickee

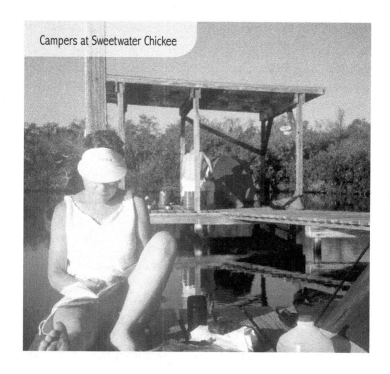

understand why Watson settled this spot on the Chatham, with views up and down the river and a deepwater dockage. Later, memoirist Totch Brown and his family would live here, fixing up the old Watson house (no longer in existence) and refurbishing the old syrup kettle and cane operations.

You can explore the site, with its syrup kettle, cistern, rusty farm equipment, foundations of the old buildings, and invasive Brazilian pepper trees that surround the area with a tangle of roots and trunks.

Holly's journal entry: *There has been no better way for me to understand the scourge of Brazilian pepper than to try to work my way through its tangled roots and limbs in my attempt today to explore the remains of Watson's homestead.*

WILLY WILLY (ground site)

Map Locator: Sections 10/L (page 84) & 11/K (page 87)
Maximum number of people: 10
Maximum number of parties: 3
Maximum number of nights: 3
Facilities: Dock, privy, & 2 picnic tables

▶ According to Larry Perez in his book *Words in the Wilderness,* this site was named for the Seminole Willy Willy, who camped in this area.

This spot is ideal for motorboaters, and if the site is crowded, you may have to pull your boat to the shore on either side of the small dock, where the mud is rather solid and will not bog you down. In a clearing surrounded by hammock vegetation, campsites are close together. A weekday visit may give you a better chance at solitude, but it's no guarantee.

From the tent at Jewell Key

Among the understory plants here, you will find the small-leaved white indigoberry, along with ferns. In the evening, you may see fireflies flickering. The water here is quite fresh, and you might spot alligators cruising nearby.

Anne's journal entry: *Paddling here today, I enjoyed seeing wood storks sailing over us—never many, just one or two at a time. And one intense roseate spoonbill against the blue sky.*

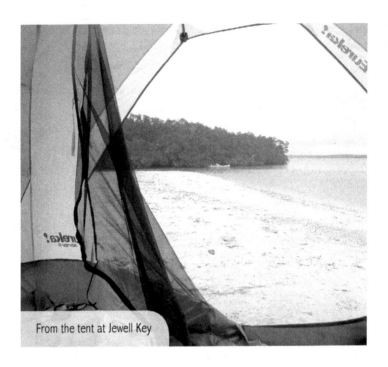

Part Six: Everglades Flora, Fauna, People, & Places

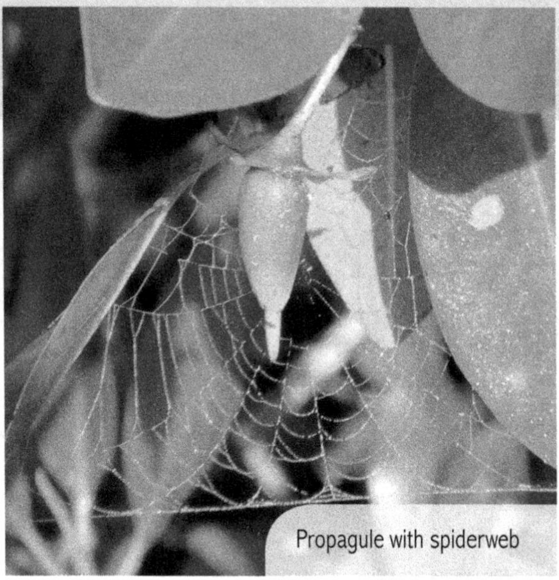

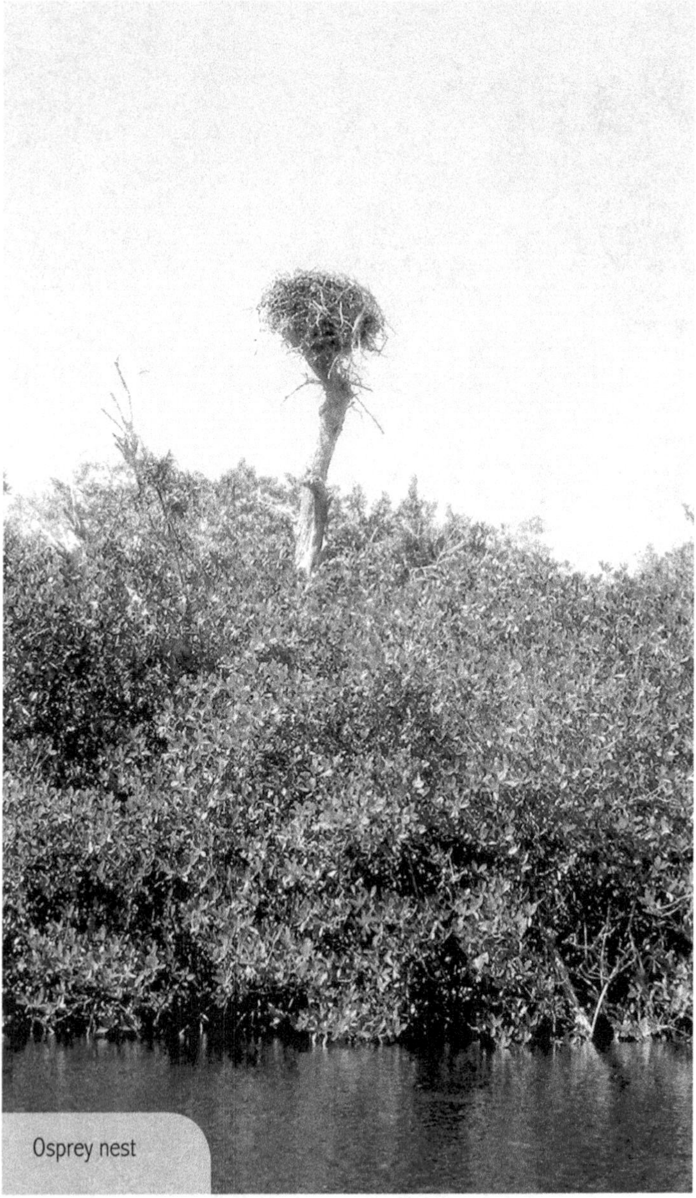

Osprey nest

There is plenty to be curious about when paddling the areas we describe. "Where did this river get its name?" or "What is this fish that's trying to jump into my boat?" In these pages, where topics are listed in alphabetical order, you may find your answer. Here, we offer small bits of information about some of the flora and fauna, as well as the human history, that you may encounter or wonder about along your route. Then, if you're still curious, you may want to consult Appendix 6, Suggested Reading, on page 283, and learn more when you return home.

Note: If an item in this glossary is specific to a particular paddling locale described elsewhere in this guidebook, we provide a cross-reference.

AMERICAN ALLIGATOR

Alligator mississippiensis lives in fresh water but can travel through brackish and occasionally salt water. The Spanish called the animal *el lagarto*, meaning "the lizard." You may distinguish the alligator from its American crocodile cousin by the alligator's rounded snout and nearly black color (see next entry for comparative features).

AMERICAN CROCODILE

Crocodylus acutus can tolerate fresh, brackish, or salt water but prefers salt. The Everglades is the only place in the world where crocodiles and alligators can sometimes be seen in the same body of water. You are most likely to spot the American crocodile on the Buttonwood Canal near the Flamingo Marina. While their numbers are said to be increasing, viewing this endangered species remains a rare opportunity. Unlike the American alligator, crocodile snouts are elongated, and their bodies are gray.

Many of the world's species of crocodile, as dramatically depicted on TV, are aggressive attackers. The American crocodile is a more docile species, even somewhat shy.

BROMELIAD

A relative of pineapple and Spanish moss, *Tillandsia* is the bromeliad genus you will see perched in the trees, particularly along narrower waterways.

These air plants attach to trees but are not parasitic. Instead, holding rain in the cups of their leaves, they take their food from the nutritious soup of rainwater that drips down from the host tree canopy. Salamanders, snakes, lizards, insects, and snails all drink from the bromeliad's natural reservoirs, and some lay their eggs there or even take up residence.

BUTTONWOOD

You can expect to see this tree throughout your paddles. Named for its spherical flowers and fruit, buttonwood (*Conocarpus erectus*) grows in association with mangroves. You can spot the buttonwoods among the mangroves by observing their narrower leaves, often with scatterings of reddish leaves among the green and yellow. Dead buttonwoods display beautiful, often twisting forms, sometimes bleached almost white by the sun. For a time there was a thriving industry in the Everglades that cut buttonwood for firewood or burned it to make charcoal, and buttonwood branches have often been sold as driftwood in the tourist trade.

BUTTONWOOD CANAL

In order to provide a water connection between Flamingo and Whitewater Bay, the Buttonwood Canal was dredged from limestone bedrock in 1956 and 1957. However, because of the negative environmental impact of salt water coming up the canal into Whitewater Bay, a dam (called "The Plug") was built in 1982 near the Flamingo Marina. The dam prevents direct travel from the canal into Florida Bay.

CABBAGE ISLAND

Located near the Rodgers River Chickee (see page 235), this island was named for its cabbage palms, also called sabal palms (*Sabal palmetto*). It is one of the few palms native to Florida and is the Florida state tree. The cabbage palm provided a source of food for early pioneers. Its heart, or bud, is still eaten today, but cutting it out kills the palm.

CALUSA

Known as the "fierce people," the Calusa inhabited southwest Florida for approximately 2,000 years. Unlike other Native Americans of Florida, they rarely hunted or farmed; rather, they lived primarily off the rich bounty of the sea, creating sizable middens from immense numbers of mollusk shells. They dug canals, built seawalls, wove fish traps, fashioned pottery, and crafted intricate wooden masks and carvings of deer, alligators, and panthers. Evidence of this early culture was recorded in a 1575 written account of the Spanish shipwreck survivor Hernando d'Escalante Fontaneda, who lived with the Calusa for 17 years. Following the European arrival, the Calusa were decimated by diseases, such as smallpox and measles, from which they had no immunity, and they were attacked by Creek raiders; the "fierce people" disappeared from Florida by the mid-18th century. Current archeological digs continue the investigation into the fascinating Calusa culture.

CHEVELIER BAY

Jean Chevelier, who lived for a time near the bay that bears his name (see pages 68 and 72), was the most famous of the Everglades plumers, who hunted birds for their feathers. Some of his specimens made it to museums. In one season he was reported to have brought in 11,000 skins and plumes of Florida birds. Known as "Old Frenchman," he may have come from France, though others believe he hailed from Montreal. In addition to pluming, he hunted for lost Spanish gold and is reported to have left buried treasure on one of the islands, but no one has ever been able to find it.

CHICKEE

The Calusa people were the first to create these open-sided, cypress log frames with palmetto thatched roofs. Later, Seminoles built them for use as homes or shelters on the hammocks and islands of the Everglades. The word *chickee* means "house," and chickees historically functioned as sleeping, cooking, and eating platforms—as do the contemporary versions, constructed for today's paddlers.

CHOKOLOSKEE ISLAND

For more than 4,000 years, Chokoloskee was home to the Native Americans of the Glades culture, then to the Calusa. Constructed by these early inhabitants from millions of empty mollusk shells, the island rises 20 feet above sea level, is 10 miles long, and is about 2 miles wide. Its name comes from Seminole words meaning "old house."

In the 1870s, several U.S. Civil War veterans settled in Chokoloskee, and in 1886 C. G. McKinney came in search of good health. When he petitioned for a post office, he called the place Comfort. But within a year it was decided that Comfort was a poor name for a place with so many "swamp angels" (mosquitoes), and it became Chokoloskee.

After a century of a fishing, farming, and trading economy, traditional sources of income became less available in the 1970s and 1980s. Enterprising residents turned to marijuana smuggling, and for a time enjoyed quite a reputation for their talents. Today Chokoloskee is a quiet place, a destination for fishermen and crabbers. Many of the locals are knowledgeable guides, and eco-tourism is rapidly becoming a main source of income.

COOT

American coots (*Fulica americana*) are dark-gray swimming birds with white bills and lobed toes (rather than webbed feet), and they resemble ducks. They congregate in groups called rafts and feed on vegetation that grows in fresh water. Unfortunately, construction of the Buttonwood Canal in 1956–57 caused an infusion of salt water into Coot Bay, and the great rafts of coot are gone. Lesser numbers do appear in the Glades, and Coot Bay still carries their name.

CUTHBERT LAKE

If you embark on the overnight South Everglades outing West Lake to Alligator Creek (see page 195), you will pass close to Cuthbert Lake, important in Everglades ecological history.

In 1903 Guy Bradley, the newly appointed game warden for the Everglades, led Arthur Cleveland Bent and the Reverend Herbert K. Job through narrow mangrove channels and open lakes to Cuthbert Lake to view Cuthbert Lake Rookery.

Bent described it this way in his *Life Histories of North American Marsh Birds*: "The afternoon was well spent when we emerged on the open waters of Cuthbert Lake and saw ahead of us the object of our search, a mangrove island, about a mile distant, literally covered with birds. It was a beautiful sight as the afternoon sun shone full upon it; hundreds of white and blue herons, and a score or two of beautiful 'pink curlews' could be plainly seen against the dark green of the mangroves, like feathered gems on a cushion of green velvet."

But by 1904, Cuthbert Rookery had been "shot out" by plume hunters. In 1905 Bradley was himself shot dead in the line of duty, as described in the Johnson Key excursion, on page 183.

DOLPHIN

Although bottlenose dolphins (*Tursiops truncates*) are saltwater mammals, you are apt to see them on most paddle routes described in this book.

As members of the Cetacea family, dolphins are small whales and, like their larger cousins, travel and fish in groups called pods. They locate their prey by emitting sounds (echolocation) through their blowholes, and they also vocalize and use body language (leaps and tail slaps) to communicate with one another. If you get a sense that they are observing or interacting with you, you are probably right, as they are intelligent and curious creatures. Their diet consists primarily of fish, shrimp, squid, and crabs, and you may see them herding such prey up onto mudbanks.

FLAMINGO

After first considering End of the World as a name, the six families who lived here in 1893 chose Flamingo. While that distinctive namesake bird is not native to Florida, flocks visited the area from their natural range in Cuba and the Bahamas.

At the town's height, around the turn of the 20th century, 50 families lived in Flamingo, and they fished, farmed, and made buttonwood charcoal for trade in Key West. After Everglades National Park was established in 1947, Flamingo's few remaining residents were relocated, and now the area serves as a gateway to the Wilderness Waterway and Florida Bay.

In 1959 a 103-room hotel opened and became a popular lodging destination for visitors to the park until the lodge and cabins were destroyed by Hurricanes Katrina and Wilma in 2005. As of this writing, the National Park Service (NPS) has plans for rebuilding facilities, and a café is open for business.

GUMBO LIMBO

Look for this stout-limbed tree on the Bear Lake Canoe Trail (see page 159) or on Sandfly Island (see page 129).

"You can take a limb of it and plant it as a fence post and it will grow," reports Rob Storter in his memoir, *Crackers in the Glade*. Known for its copper-colored, flaky bark, the gumbo limbo (*Bursera simaruba*) is often called the "tourist tree," reminiscent of the red, peeling, sunburned skin of Florida's visitors. Gumbo limbos can be found throughout the Caribbean and deep south Florida. The Haitian people make drums from the wood, and in the United States, carousel horses were traditionally carved from gumbo limbo. The resin is used for varnish, glue, incense, car air fresheners, and, historically, to treat gout.

HAMMOCK

If you find yourself in a place that is slightly elevated from surrounding wetlands, where broad-leaved hardwood trees create shade for a complex understory, where bromeliads perch and hang in branches, and where ferns grow from the damp duff, you can be sure that you are in a tropical hardwood hammock.

Most of the trees in deep south Florida hammocks are of West Indian origin, their seeds having floated on the waves, flown with hurricane winds, or ridden in the bellies of birds. Gumbo limbos, mahoganies, pigeon plums, and wild tamarinds mix with oaks and cabbage palms. If you smell a musky (some say skunky) scent, you are in the presence of white stoppers, an almost omnipresent hammock understory tree. These hammocks (also spelled hummocks) are preferred residences of barred owls. Listen for their "who-cooks-for-you?" call from the canopy. Hammocks have given refuge to wildlife and humans alike through the centuries. Noble Hammock (see page 175) offers a fine example.

HARNEY RIVER

Serving in Florida during the Seminole Wars, Lieutenant Colonel William S. Harney tracked the Seminoles deeper into the Glades than white men had previously managed to do. In 1840 he followed the war chief Chekika to his hiding place. Harney commanded his force to dress and paint themselves as Seminole warriors. They conducted a surprise attack, killing Chekika and capturing many of his band. All of those captured were hung. Returning to Fort Dallas, Harney intended to lead his men along an easier route than the one they had taken into the Everglades. His intent was to take Shark River to the Gulf, but he missed the turnoff, discovering another route, the river that is now called Harney.

IBIS

Probing the mudflats with their long, down-curving bills, the American white ibis (*Eudocimus albus* and pronounced "EYE-bis") search for frogs and crustaceans. The adults are white with black wingtips visible in flight, while the juveniles are brown or splotched brown and white with a white belly. After feeding in various places during the day, chains of ibis fly back to join others to roost for the night. The noted biologist Archie Carr wrote in his book *The Everglades,* "As the little, dark green islands received their birds they flowered, as if with magnolia blooms."

LIMESTONE

A sedimentary rock made of calcium carbonate, limestone formed as billions of seashells and other plant and animal parts fell to the seafloor and coalesced. Underlying most of the Wilderness Waterway, the Tamiami Limestone Formation, laid down 6 million years ago, is the oldest of the six formations of south Florida. Near Flamingo, the 1956-57 construction of the Buttonwood Canal (see page 246) exposed areas of bedrock that are part of the Miami Formation, which is younger, at about 100,000 years old. You will also see limestone under the water on the Nine Mile Pond day trip (see page 171).

MANATEE

Formally named the West Indian manatee, *Trichechus manatus* swims near the mouths of the Everglades rivers, in Chokoloskee Bay, and in the Gulf. Watch for the spots, called footprints, that are created by the paddle stroke of their tails. As slow-moving creatures, manatees are frequently injured or killed in encounters with boat propellers. Like elephants, their close relative, manatees are vegetarians. While you are paddling on the water's surface, they are grazing beneath you on 60–100 pounds of water plants each day.

MANGROVE

Mangrove comes from the word for "mangle" in the language of the Arawak people, who were natives of the Caribbean. In the Everglades, the mangrove ecosystem is amazingly productive, with its constant "rain" of vegetation. In addition to providing shelter and food for marine organisms, the mangrove tangle (sometimes called a mangle) afforded shelter for Seminoles and settlers during hurricanes.

Three different types—red, black, and white—live in the Glades. Those closest to, and actually in, salt water are the red mangroves, *Rhizophora mangle*. Their arching prop roots and spreading growth habit led the Seminoles to call them "walking trees." Red mangroves also send down aerial roots, hanging from the branches like vines, until they reach the ground and become rooted. The red mangrove has yellow waxy flowers, with seeds that germinate before they leave the tree and become those "string bean" propagules (seeds) that drop and float off to start new mangrove islands.

The black mangrove, *Avicennia germinans*, sends up pencil-like breathing tubes called pneumatophores. Black mangroves can tolerate the tide rising regularly above those tubes but cannot survive prolonged submersion. Their leaves secrete salt water and taste salty if you lick them. You can spot the black mangroves by their slightly gray-green leaves.

The tallest of the mangroves, white mangroves (*Laguncularia racemosa*), grow farther from the water, on higher ground. In 1960 Hurricane Donna destroyed 50%–75% of the mature mangroves along the Everglades's Shark River, one of the tallest stands of mangroves in the world. There are still some tall white mangroves along the Shark River—to an extent that you almost have a sense of paddling through a valley.

MOSQUITO

You will encounter "swamp angels" just about anywhere in the Everglades, primarily in the evenings. The good news is that while there are 43 species of mosquitoes in South Florida, only 13 species bite. And it's just the female that bites, using your blood protein to produce her eggs.

History relates some ingenious mosquito repellents: the Seminoles coated their skin with fish oil or mud. Both Seminoles and pioneers burned black mangrove wood in smudge pots, producing smoke to thwart the insects. And palmetto leaves made excellent fans for dispelling the creatures. In Flamingo, settlers' houses had an entry room called the loser where people brushed themselves off to "lose" mosquitoes. For more modern tips on dealing with mosquitoes, see "Insects," on page 204.

As annoying as mosquitoes can be, they serve vital functions in the ecosystem. Their larvae, which grow in water, are food for small fish, which in turn are food for larger fish. Adult mosquitoes are prey for bats, frogs, insects, birds, and lizards.

MULLET

What is that fish that looks like it will jump right into your boat? It's a striped mullet (*Mugil cephalus*). Why this torpedo-shaped fish jumps is subject to speculation: To avoid predators? To rid themselves of parasites? To communicate with fellow mullet? For aerial respiration? To clear their gills of mud? To rid themselves of gas? Because they are happy? Scientists still don't know the answer.

Mullet feed on algae and decaying plant and animal matter called marine snow, and they are a major food source for other saltwater fish and for the Atlantic bottlenose dolphin. The latter catch them by "fish kicking," hitting the fish with their tail flukes and tossing them into the air. Humans catch them with cast nets, as this fish shuns baited hooks.

NICKERBEAN & NICKERNUT

You will surely see the thorny nickerbean vine, *Caesalpinia bonduc,* at the Picnic Key Campsite (see page 233). The vine produces two seeds, or nickernuts, in each of its prickly pods. Smooth, round, and luminous, these seeds are called sea pearls. Named after

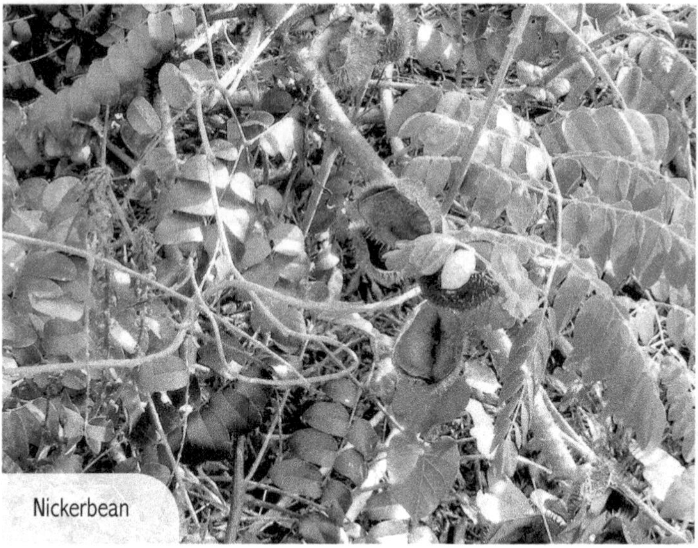
Nickerbean

a Dutch clay marble, a nickernut is quite durable and buoyant and can survive months at sea, sprouting in soft sand where it lands. On Caribbean islands and in Mexico, nickernuts are strung as bracelets, necklaces, and rosaries, and they are used as tokens in a game called oware, an island version of the game mancala. Pioneer children of South Florida sometimes used the seeds as marbles.

THE NIGHTMARE

No one seems to know exactly when or how The Nightmare got its name. This narrow, winding route between the Broad River and the Harney River, connecting the north and south channels of the Glades, was not named at all on maps in William G. Truesdell's first edition (1969) or second edition (1985) of the *Guide to the Wilderness Waterway*. It appears now, however, on both NOAA and Waterproof charts, and the name has entered the historical lore of Waterway paddlers.

It was in the mid-1960s that ranger Richard "Dick" Stokes spearheaded the search for an inland passage that would link north and south. After several failed attempts, he and his fellow searchers finally located a barely passable channel. Following his retirement in 1981, Stokes wrote an open letter to the media, in which he said: "As far as I could find out, none of the locals had ever been through this waterway. No one knew of it nor did it show on any of the modern navigation charts. There was no sign of the creek ever being used within modern times. I strongly suspect that the only use was by the Calusa."

ONION KEY

Paddling the Wilderness Waterway section 8/N (see page 78), you will pass the key that local memoirist Totch Brown claims was named by settler Gregorio Lopez because he ate his last onion here. In another story, related in historian Charlton Tebeau's *Man in the Everglades*, an unidentified man chose this solitary spot to homestead with his wife and grow onions. In its earliest known human history, the key was a Calusa settlement. In 1925 the key became the field headquarters for the real estate development company Poinciana Mainland, and later still, an NPS wilderness campsite. After a multistoried past, the key is now off-limits to the public.

OSPREY

Also known as fish hawks, *Pandion haliaetus* build massive stick nests on the tops of poles or trees, and you are likely to see them anywhere in your paddles. You might hear their "kee-uk" call and see them dive to grab fish from the water with their powerful talons. After catching a fish and resuming flight, the osprey turns the prey's head forward, avoiding drag.

OYSTER

Eastern, or Atlantic, oysters (*Crassostrea virginica*) are bivalve filter feeders that settle on sandbars and create oyster beds that lie across the current. As the oyster colony is bathed in the incoming tide, a tube called a siphon sucks in nutrients from the water. Oysters trap sediment, which gives mangrove propagules (long, string bean–shaped seeds) a place to anchor and form new mangrove islands. They are also an important food source for birds, fish, and marine invertebrates. In short, oysters are a keystone species, cleaning water, stabilizing shorelines, and playing vital roles in the complexity of the Everglades ecosystem.

PLATE CREEK

You will paddle this creek on Wilderness Waterway section 7/O (see page 75). Local memoirist Totch Brown, whose tales of the Everglades capture much of settler history, tells the story that the 19th-century settler and river namesake Gregorio Lopez named this creek when he lost a plate in the water here. (Yes, it's reminiscent of Señor Lopez's last onion on Onion Key, as described previously.)

RODGERS RIVER (BAY)

Rodgers River was named for Colonel S. St. George Rodgers, a member of the Florida Mounted Volunteers in the Third Seminole War, who traveled with 110 men from Fort Myers to what he called Chokoliska Key in 1857. You'll paddle the Waterway here in sections 10/L and 11/K (see pages 83 and 86), and may stay at the Rodgers River Chickee (see page 235). At the turn of the 20th century, several pioneer families were established along Rodgers River, but now all the homesteads are gone and you are in the heart of the wilderness, surrounded by bays and the ever-present mangroves.

ROSEATE SPOONBILL

If you see a pink bird flying overhead, chances are that it is a roseate spoonbill (*Ajaia ajaja*), not the nonnative flamingo. If you see a number of these birds, you may notice that some are pinker than others. The degree of pink depends upon age and diet. For the first 2 years, roseate spoonbills are quite white. In adults, the pink color is enhanced when their diet is rich in shrimp and other crustaceans. During the plume rage of the early 20th century, these birds were prized for their colorful feathers. Whole wings were used to make fashionable feather fans.

At the water's edge, spoonbills sweep their flattish bills, filtering out small food items from the water. Like their ibis relatives, roseate spoonbills fly with necks outstretched and with rapid wing beats. Watch for their startling beauty as you paddle various Everglades routes, and look for them at Alligator Creek Campsite (see page 214).

SEAGRASS

Seagrass meadows waving in the clear waters of Florida Bay constitute an extremely productive ecosystem. Two types of seagrass predominate here: the broad-leaved turtle grass (*Thalassia testudinum*) and the cylindrical manatee grass (*Syringodium filiforme*). Many marine species feed on seagrass, its detritus, or the single-celled algae that grow on its leaves; other marine species take shelter among its blades or prey on the animals that feed or hide in these meadows. The meadows also serve as nurseries for many sport and commercial fish and for other marine life important to Florida's economy. In addition, seagrass stabilizes the seabed and helps maintain water clarity by filtering debris. The grass releases oxygen into the water so quickly that one can see air bubbles escaping from its leaves. Enjoy the seagrass vistas out in Florida Bay.

SEMINOLE & MICCOSUKEE

Following the Creek War of 1813-14, the Seminoles (who called themselves the "free people") moved south from Georgia into northern Florida. After the Florida territory was transferred from Spain to the U.S. in 1821, a series of three Seminole Wars (1835–1858) drove the "free people" deeper south into the Everglades. Although many were killed, captured, or forced to move west to Arkansas, about 100 Seminoles remained in the Glades, never having signed a peace treaty with the U.S. Their descendents live here today on reservation land and maintain their tribal culture and traditions. A separate tribe, the Miccosukee, separated from the Seminoles, forming their own tribal government on lands just north of Everglades National Park.

SHARK RIVER

The Shark River Slough (pronounced "slew") is a wide wetland depression that carries fresh water in its slow flow southwest through the Everglades to the Gulf of Mexico. One of the primary channels that this water takes as it nears the Gulf is the Shark River. The land along the Shark is very low, and there have been few attempts to homestead along this river. In the early 20th century, the Manetta Company did try operations for extracting tannic acid and lumber from the mangrove forests, but the business ceased when a 1920 Category 4 hurricane destroyed its structures. Yes, bull and hammerhead sharks do visit the Shark River.

SMALLWOOD STORE

C. S. "Ted" Smallwood settled on Chokoloskee Island in the 1890s. He farmed in his early years, including the first few years after he married his neighbor's daughter, Mamie House. Then the couple opened a store in their home to supplement their income. They saved up money until they could afford to buy lumber, and Smallwood built a trading post. In 1906 he became postmaster, with the post office inside the store, and eventually passed that position on to his daughter Thelma.

That first store was built on ground level at the water's edge but was severely damaged by a hurricane in 1924. Smallwood rebuilt, elevating the store on high pilings. Since then, the Historic Smallwood Store has weathered multiple hurricanes. Placed on the National Register of Historic Places in 1974, the store is now a museum, still under the auspices of the Smallwood family.

SNOWY EGRET

You will see *Egretta thula* almost anywhere on Everglades adventures. Easily identified by their black legs and bright yellow feet (often referred to as "golden slippers"), snowy egrets are small, all-white-bodied herons that feed throughout the Everglades and along the Gulf shore. These birds sometimes use their golden feet as fishing lures, flying over the water and skipping their "slippers" to entice fish to the surface, where the egrets then can snatch them with their beaks. Snowy egrets were almost hunted to extinction for their aigrettes, the spectacular lacy plumes they display during breeding season. Their populations have not fully recovered, but numbers have increased considerably.

SWALLOW-TAILED KITE

Soaring above the Waterway with distinctive V-shaped tails, swallow-tailed kites (*Elanoides forficatus*) are raptors. As hawks, they capture insects, snakes, and lizards out of the air and the treetops while in flight. They have been known to snatch up a nest with baby birds and, holding the nest like a drinking bowl, consume the contents. They are constant fliers, rarely landing except to nest. Energy-efficient, they seldom flap their wings, but rotate their tails to turn as they drift in the air currents. Because they are migratory, you are likely to see them only February–August.

TABANIDAE (Yellow Flies)

Yellow flies, particularly notorious in Florida for their biting power, can set your arms and ankles stinging wildly. But deerflies and horseflies give a mean bite too. Be alert for the entire Tabanidae (pronounced "tah-BAN-ni-dee") clan, particularly in the hours around sunrise and sunset and when the air is still.

Especially watch for them in the shade, where these flies tend to lurk. They locate prey primarily by sight and are drawn to dark colors, but they also recognize prey by scent. You can make yourself less attractive to them by wearing light clothes and scenting yourself with lemon eucalyptus oil or other insect repellent. But keep the Benadryl cream handy.

Although these species are similar in appearance, yellow flies are more golden yellow than the other two, and horseflies are a little larger than either yellow flies or deerflies. Sometimes, however, all of these are referred to locally as deerflies.

TABBY

Known as coastal concrete, tabby is made of equal parts lime, oyster shell, sand, and water. The mixture is poured into molds and hardens into a building material that is extremely durable. Weather-strong, it was often the building material of choice in pioneer southwest Florida. Tabby fragments of homes, cisterns, and other structures remain as evidence of human habitation on a number of islands along the Waterway, including Lopez River Campsite, Darwin's Place, and The Watson Place (see pages 230, 219, and 239, respectively).

TARPON

Known as the "silver king" in Florida waters, tarpon (*Megalops atlanticus*) are primarily inshore fish. They feature silver sides covered with large scales, and they have a modified swim bladder that enables them to gulp air at the surface. In addition, they have a short dorsal fin with a threadlike trailing edge, but when they swim near the surface, the tail sticks out of the water and can resemble a second fin. Tarpon feed both day and night, and they spawn offshore May–October.

TURNER RIVER

Captain Richard Turner, a U.S. Army Seminole War scout, guided an expedition up "Chokolisca Creek" in 1857. In 1871 he returned to establish a homestead on a Calusa shell mound 0.25 mile up what is now known as the Turner River. He and several other families farmed there for a number of years.

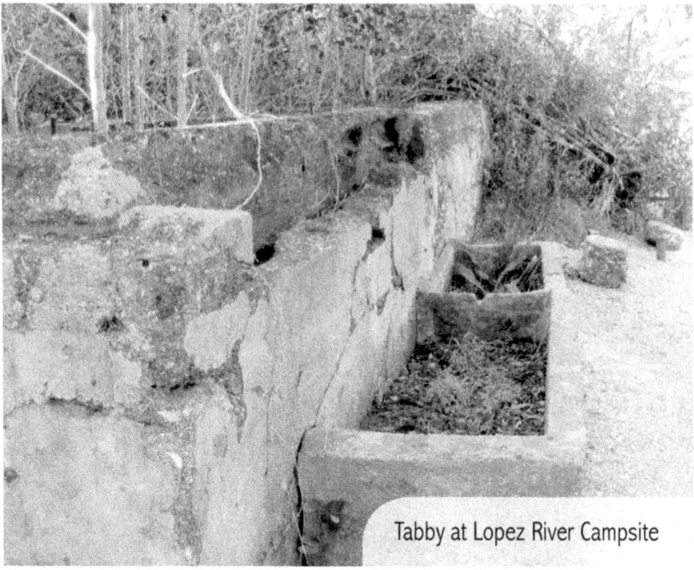

Tabby at Lopez River Campsite

When you paddle the Halfway Creek/Turner River Loop (see page 122), look for regular rows of mounds constructed perpendicular to the riverbanks and extending 0.5 mile away from the channel. Due to heavy subtropical vegetation, it may not be easy to see them from a kayak or canoe, but you may be able to spot them if you look behind the mangroves. If you miss them, know that they are there and that you're paddling through a place where ancient, and then pioneering, people had a thriving culture.

WORM ROCK

Often confused with corals or with the Sabellariid worm reefs that lie off Florida's Atlantic Coast, worm rock is a strong structure created by snails—not by coral or by worms. One such worm rock reef can be found off the Picnic Key and Tiger Key area. Known as the worm snail (*Petaloconchus varians*), this mollusk attaches itself to a hard substrate and forms a wormlike shell that twists and coils, interlacing with the shells of thousands of other gastropods to form extensive rocklike reefs. Although worm snails are still present in the Gulf, they are no longer forming new reefs.

Appendixes

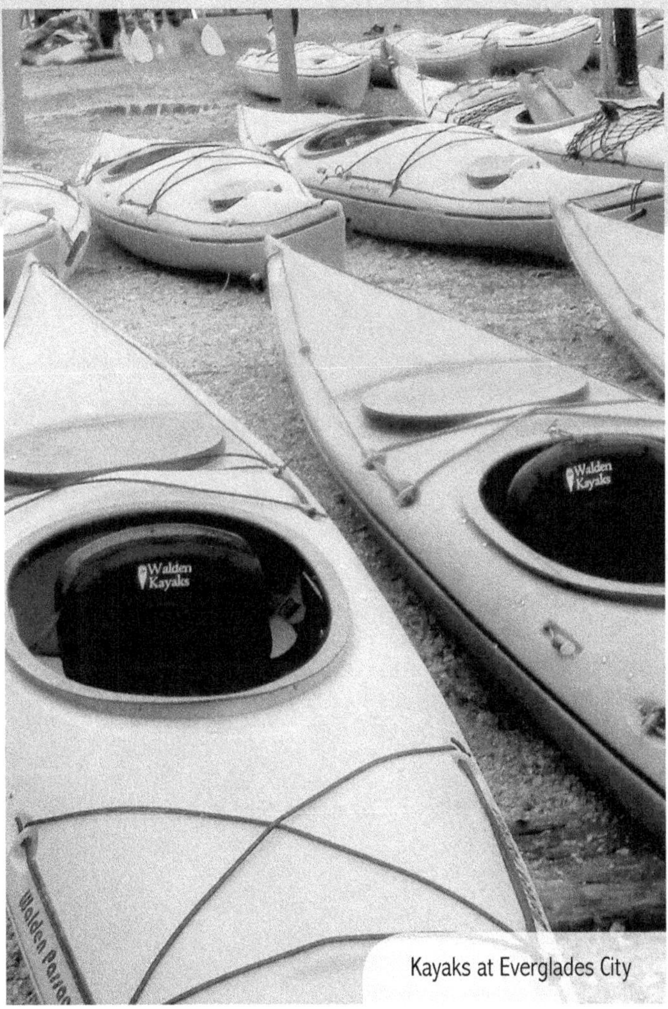

Kayaks at Everglades City

APPENDIX 1: CHECKLIST

CAMPING SUPPLIES

- Freestanding tent
- Sleeping pad
- Sleeping bag
- Camp pillow

PADDLING SUPPLIES

- Paddles (and spares)
- Wearable personal flotation device (PFD) for each person
- Whistle for each person (attached to PFD)
- Flares (recommended)
- Anchor (recommended)
- Manual water pump, or a bailer made from a gallon jug
- Sponge
- Bow and stern lights, if paddling at night
- Camp chairs (recommended)
- Ropes
- Tarp
- Bungee cords (to secure the tarp to a canoe or to attach the tent to the chickee posts)
- Dry bags
- Navigation charts
- GPS unit (optional)
- Compass
- Tide charts
- Watch, for calculating tides
- Binoculars
- Marine radio
- Long-beam flashlight (optional)

CLOTHING

- Paddling gloves
- Wide-brimmed hat
- Short-sleeved shirts or tank tops
- Long-sleeved shirt
- Quick-drying shorts
- Long pants
- Water shoes or sneakers
- Underwear
- Polypropylene long underwear (in winter)
- Socks
- Rain jacket
- Fleece jacket
- Bandannas
- Head net for insects
- Bug suit (in summer)
- Bag for dirty clothes

FOOD & WATER SUPPLIES

1 gallon of water per person per day (more in summer)

Raccoon-proof storage containers

Individual water bottle or hydration pack

Cooler (optional)

Written food plan for each day

Food for breakfast, snack, lunch, and dinner (see "Food" on page 47)

Extra day's supply of food

Small "kitchen" tarp

Stove

Propane or other fuel

Lighters

Matches in a waterproof container

Cook kit, such as nested pots with lids used as frypans

Stirring spoon, spatula, and paring knife

Bowl/plate for each person

Knife, fork, and spoon for each person

Insulated beverage cup for each person

Single-cup drip coffeemaker, or funnel (optional)

Coffee filters (optional)

Scrubbie

Biodegradable soap

Camp towel

Fishing gear and tackle (optional) and a Florida fishing license

Zip-top plastic bags for garbage

PERSONAL ITEMS

Sunglasses, with strap

Insect repellent (several for a group)

Sunscreen

Lip balm

Toilet paper

Trowel (for sites with no privy)

Hand sanitizer

Sanitary items

Prescription medications

Ibuprofen (for aches)

Antibiotic ointment (such as Neosporin, for cuts)

Diphenhydramine (such as Benadryl, for itchy insect bites)

Band-Aids

Toothbrush

Toothpaste

Floss

Deodorant

Premoistened towelettes

Nail clippers and nail file

Headlamp (and extra batteries)

APPENDIX 1: CHECKLIST (cont'd)

RECOMMENDED

Journal and/or sketchbook
Pens, or pencils with a sharpener
Camera (and extra batteries)
Reading material
Field guides (choose carefully, with size and weight in mind)
This book!

APPENDIX 2: LAUNCH SITES

EVERGLADES CITY & CHOKOLOSKEE AREA

All of the paddles out of Everglades City described in this book launch from the Gulf Coast Visitor Center of Everglades National Park. There is no launch fee. However, if launching at low tide, if you have time limitations, or for other considerations, you may wish to choose an alternative site. Each of the launch possibilities listed below also offers additional services, which are described briefly. Check websites and call sites directly for additional details, including pricing.

CHOKOLOSKEE ISLAND PARK & MARINA

1150 Hamilton Ln.
Chokoloskee, FL 34138
(239) 695-2414
chokoloskee.com

▶ Managers Wayne Schefer and Lynda Schoonover offer services not only for paddlers who launch from their floating dock but also for paddlers just passing by. For a small fee, you can paddle up and take a shower at the end of a long journey or even do your laundry. If you launch here, parking is free for day trips. Also, if you do plan to launch and land here or nearby, you can pitch a tent or rent an efficiency unit for a night.

The shop at the office is small, but you'll find ice, soft drinks, shirts, and—for those who are fishing as well as paddling—light tackle and bait. If you're in the mood for a little local reading, you can purchase a book by an author who resides in Everglades National Park, and there's a possibility you'll find a special event in progress next door at the waterside chickee. Chokoloskee Island

Park & Marina is located on the southwest side of the island.

If this is your first time out and you'd like a guide, Wayne and Lynda can help you set that up with Everglades Area Tours or a private fishing guide. The website above offers photos and information, including rate schedules for tent camping, lodging, and launching.

CHOKOLOSKEE ISLAND RESORT & MARINA

FL 29 South (Smallwood Drive;
look left immediately upon entering Chokoloskee)
Chokoloskee Island, FL 34138
(239) 695-3788
outdoor-resorts.com/ci

▶ Looking at the website, you might not be able to tell that there is a canoe and kayak launch here. You also might not realize that Kenny Brown, who started working in the family business after school when he was 6 or 7, is available to pore over the charts with you, get you oriented, and tell you some good stories about the area.

The business has changed names several times, but it's been in the same place since the 1950s. Brown's ancestors, arriving in Miami in 1859, were among the first to settle in Chokoloskee after the Civil War. He is kin to "just about everybody here," he says, and he has the genealogical charts to prove it. (Memoirist Totch Brown, mentioned throughout this guide, is one of Kenny Brown's more famous cousins.)

The company's paddle-craft launch, a discreet beach opening in the mangroves, offers an easy slide into the water. Short- or long-term parking is available near the launch. The parking fee includes trash disposal and use of the boat-rinsing station and restrooms. Fees are reduced for groups. The small bait-and-tackle shop near the road sells ice, Styrofoam coolers, bottled water, snacks, sunscreen, insect repellent, zip-top plastic bags, and hot coffee. Waterproof Charts are available, as well as a free map for day-trippers who don't want to purchase the charts.

EVERGLADES NATIONAL PARK BOAT TOURS

815 SW Copeland Ave.
Everglades City, FL 34139
(239) 695-2591

▶ Located on the same property as the Gulf Coast Visitor Center, this is an official concessionaire of Everglades National Park. Brenda Hamilton claims, "We have the cheapest canoe and kayak rentals in the whole state of Florida." In addition to canoe and kayak rentals, the shop sells both NOAA nautical charts and Waterproof Charts, as well as light gear (waterproof packs, water bottles, small compasses, whistles, and so on), soft drinks, shirts, hats, and souvenirs.

GLADES HAVEN MARINA

875 S. Copeland Ave. (FL 29 S)
Everglades City, FL 34139
(239) 695-2628 (marina)
(239) 695-2746 or (239) 695-2073 (restaurant)
theevergladesflorida.com

▶ "We enjoy people, whether we're feeding them, housing them, or sending them out in a boat," says co-owner Patty Miller. Since 1984, she and Robert Miller Sr. and Bobby Miller Jr. have been expanding all of those services in their location directly across from Everglades National Park's Gulf Coast Visitor Center.

They offer canoe and kayak launches on a rubber mat spread over concrete, and rental watercraft are available. On-site, there is a convenience store, The Oyster House full-service restaurant, and a liquor store. Glades Haven offers rental duplex cabins and houses, can lodge up to 70 people, and hosts group events.

Visit the website for details about additional services, including bike rentals, food prepared for a boat trip, and a shuttle back from Flamingo if you are planning to thru-paddle the Wilderness Waterway. Glades Haven also offers airport shuttle service to and from Fort Myers, Miami, or Fort Lauderdale; advance reservations are required.

If you don't have time to thru-paddle, but you want to get deep into the Waterway, Glades Haven will boat-shuttle you and your canoe or kayak as far as you want to go, and then you can paddle back.

HISTORIC SMALLWOOD STORE

360 Mamie St.
Chokoloskee, FL 34138
(941) 695-2989

▶ In the 19th century, Chokoloskee was a busy center of commerce, receiving boat traffic from points both north and south. On the water passages now known as the Everglades Wilderness Waterway, much of the traffic was heading to or from this very spot.

Today, you can launch from the side of this old trading post perched on pilings at a historic point of Chokoloskee Island. But you must launch when the trading post is open so that you can pay the small launch fee; hours vary seasonally, so call ahead. For day trips, you can leave your car in the museum's small parking area. If launching for an overnight or the full waterway, you'll need to arrange to leave the car at the Gulf Coast Visitor Center or elsewhere.

Paddlers passing by are welcome to stop and visit the museum and store. You can buy a bottled Coke from a 1945 Coke machine, the first to appear on Chokoloskee. (It doesn't look anything like the Coke machines of today.) Bottled water is also available. Just be sure, before you go up the stairs, that you're not tracking mud and that the bottoms of your shoes are as dry as you can get them. The old boards dry slowly.

PARKWAY MOTEL & MARINA

1180 Chokoloskee Dr.
Chokoloskee, FL 34138
(239) 695-3261
parkwaymotelandmarina.com

▶ Perched at the water's edge on property that once belonged to the area's renowned Smallwood family, the Parkway Motel & Marina sits only a short walk from the Historic Smallwood Store. Parkway also touts its southerly position on the island as "the closest access to Florida's 10,000 Islands, Everglades National Park, and The Gulf of Mexico." At high tide, you can simply launch over the side of the dock here.

At low tide, you may prefer to go a short distance to a different launch, but you still might opt to spend a night before or after your paddle in the four-room motel, or in the two-bedroom, two-bath house overlooking the marina. All offer free wireless Internet. Managers Geri and Bill Shelburne are quick to invite prospective visitors to check out their ratings on Trip Advisor (**tripadvisor.com**).

In the small store at the motel office, you'll find bottled water, soft drinks, caps, shirts, and light fishing tackle. You can also arrange for guided canoe and kayak tours.

FLAMINGO

FLAMINGO MARINA

Everglades National Park

(239) 695-3101

nps.gov/planyourvisit/marinasandramps.htm

▶ If leaving for a Wilderness Waterway thru-paddle or for a paddle in Florida Bay, you will launch from the Flamingo Marina at the end of the main park road at the Homestead/Florida City entrance. Immediately adjacent to the marina store, canoe and kayak rentals are available from Everglades National Park Boat Tours II.

The store sells navigational charts, sunscreen, insect repellent, head nets, light gear, basic groceries, and ice. Store clerks post current weather conditions on a whiteboard at the checkout.

APPENDIX 3: OUTFITTERS, SUPPLIERS, & CANOE/KAYAK RENTALS

EVERGLADES CITY & CHOKOLOSKEE AREA

THE IVEY HOUSE BED AND BREAKFAST

107 Camellia St. East
Everglades City, FL 34139
(877) 567-0679 or (239) 695-3299
iveyhouse.com

▶ Canoe and kayak rental is handy at this bed-and-breakfast, which also offers eco-tours, a gift shop, and a location near the historic Everglades City business district.

NAPLES KAYAK COMPANY

11369 E. Tamiami Trl.
Naples, FL 34113
(239) 262-6149
napleskayakcompany.com

▶ In Naples, 36 miles north of Everglades City, Naples Kayak Company is a comprehensive kayak outfitter. The company sells and rents kayaks and gear, offers instruction, and leads tours.

RIGHT CHOICE SUPERMARKET

102 Buckner Ave.
Everglades City, FL 34139

▶ Here is the closest thing to a full grocery store in Everglades City and Chokoloskee. Near the traffic circle.

WIN-CAR HARDWARE

209 N. Collier Ave.
Everglades City, FL 34139
(239) 695-3201

▶ You'll find a lot more than hardware here. Shop for quality coolers and thermoses, navigational charts, cookware, books, Tilley hats, bug suits, and gear. You can also ask the folks behind the counter about local history and local resources. In many cases, you will be talking to descendants of original settlers of the area.

FLAMINGO AREA

BACKCOUNTRY COWBOY OUTFITTERS

Mile Marker 82.2, 82240 Overseas Hwy.
Islamorada, FL 33036
(305) 517-4177
backcountrycowboy.com

▶ Another comprehensive canoe and kayak outfitter, Backcountry rents boats and guides tours from Islamorada, Flamingo, and Everglades City—including Wilderness Waterway paddles.

EVERGLADES INTERNATIONAL HOSTEL & EVERGLADES TOURS

20 SW Second Ave.
Florida City, FL 33034
(800) 372-3874 or (305) 248-1122
evergladeshostel.com

▶ Welcoming to backpackers, the hostel offers overflow tent camping in the courtyard, as well as canoe and kayak rental, guided tours, custom tours, bike and rack rentals, and Wilderness Waterway shuttles.

EVERGLADES NATIONAL PARK BOAT TOURS II, INC.

Flamingo Marina at the end of the main park road
Homestead, FL 33034
(239) 695-3101

▶ Here at the marina, you can rent canoes, kayaks, and bikes. Double canoes are available for carrying up to three people, and family-size canoes hold up to four people. Rentals are available for Buttonwood Canal and Nine Mile Pond, and they will also rent for Hells Bay and overnight trips if you have your own car carrier. Narrated tours on large boats are also available for Florida Bay or backcountry.

FLORIDA BAY OUTFITTERS

104050 Overseas Hwy.
Key Largo, FL 33037
(305) 451-3018
kayakfloridakeys.com

▶ A comprehensive canoe and kayak outfitter, Florida Bay sells and rents watercraft, offers instruction, provides a Wilderness Waterway shuttle, and leads group and custom tours.

APPENDIX 4: RESOURCE OVERVIEW

Everglades City/Chokoloskee	Launch Site	Lodging or Camping	Supplies	Canoe/Kayak Rental	Wilderness Waterway Shuttle
Chokoloskee Island Park & Marina	✓	✓	✓	–	–
Chokoloskee Island Resort & Marina	✓	✓	✓	✓	–
Everglades Nat'l Park Boat Tours	✓	–	✓	✓	–
Glades Haven Marina	✓	✓	✓	✓	✓
Ivey House	–	✓	✓	–	–
Naples Kayak Company	–	–	✓	✓	–
Parkway Motel & Marina	✓	✓	✓	–	–
Right Choice Supermarket	–	–	✓	–	–
Smallwood Store	✓	–	–	–	–
Win-Car Hardware	–	–	✓	–	–

Flamingo Area	Launch Site	Lodging or Camping	Supplies	Canoe/Kayak Rental	Wilderness Waterway Shuttle
Backcountry Cowboy Outfitters	—	—	✓	✓	✓
Everglades Internat'l Hostel & Tours	—	✓	—	✓	✓
Everglades Nat'l Park Boat Tours II	✓	—	—	✓	—
Flamingo Marina	✓	—	✓	✓	—
Florida Bay Outfitters	✓	—	✓	✓	✓

APPENDIX 4 (cont'd)

TENT CAMPING

In addition to the camping possibilities noted in the charts above, there are a few choices on the Tamiami Trail (US 41) within 20 miles of the junction with FL 29 at Everglades City.

COLLIER-SEMINOLE STATE PARK

(between Naples and Everglades City)
20200 Tamiami Trl. East
Naples, FL 34114
(239) 394-3397
floridastateparks.org/collierseminole

MONUMENT LAKE CAMPGROUND, BIG CYPRESS NATIONAL PRESERVE

Open August 28–April 15
For availability, call the Oasis Visitor Center at (239) 695-1201.
Reservations not accepted
nps.gov/bicy/planyourvisit/campgrounds.htm

If launching in the south, there are two camping possibilities located in the park.

FLAMINGO CAMPGROUND, EVERGLADES NATIONAL PARK

(Homestead/Florida City entrance)
For reservations, call (877) 444-6777 after November 20.
nps.gov/ever/planyourvisit/flamcamp.htm

LONG PINE KEY CAMPGROUND, EVERGLADES NATIONAL PARK

(Homestead/Florida City entrance)
Reservations not accepted
(305) 242-7873
nps.gov/ever/planyourvisit/longpinecamp.htm

APPENDIX 5: INTERNET RESOURCES

With its typically frequent updates, the Internet is a valuable tool for Everglades-bound travelers and paddlers.

EVERGLADES INFORMATION

EVERGLADES NATIONAL PARK

Visit **nps.gov/ever** for a downloadable "Wilderness Trip Planner" and "Florida Bay Map and Guide." Find paddling information under "Plan Your Visit."

FRIENDS OF THE EVERGLADES

Visit **everglades.org** for a newsletter and activity information from this organization founded by Marjory Stoneman Douglas (see "Ecology & Environment," on page 18).

AUDUBON OF FLORIDA

Visit **fl.audubon.org** to track progress on the Everglades Restoration Plan.

PADDLING THE EVERGLADES

EVERGLADES DIARY

Visit **evergladesdiary.com** for Wilderness Waterway and campsite descriptions and photos.

EVERGLADES EXPLORATION NETWORK

Visit **gladesgodeep.ning.com,** a network for discussion of hiking, paddling, and biking into the Everglades and Big Cypress National Preserve.

FLORIDA PADDLING TRAILS ASSOCIATION

Visit **floridapaddlingtrails.com** to view recent waterway reports on the Everglades and Florida Bay.

NAVIGATIONAL MAPS & CHARTS

NOAA NAUTICAL CHARTS

Visit **nauticalcharts.noaa.gov** for paper charts for all sections of the Wilderness Waterway.

WATERPROOF CHARTS

Visit **waterproofcharts.com** for Waterproof Charts for all sections of the Wilderness Waterway.

USGS QUADRANGLES

Visit **usgs.gov/pubprod** to order 7.5-minute quadrangles. Visit **edcsns17.cr.usgs.gov/NewEarthExplorer** to determine Everglades quadrangles.

WEATHER & TIDE CHARTS

Visit **weather.com** for current and 10-day forecasts from The Weather Channel.

Visit **saltwatertides.com** for high- and low-tide times according to location and date.

APPENDIX 6: SUGGESTED READING

NATURE AND POLITICS

Carr, Archie Farley. *The Everglades.* New York: Time/Life Books, 1973. Rich with photographs and a literary style, this volume is out of print, but used copies are available. Time/Life's American Wilderness series' author is a noted biologist, who leads us through the various ecosystems of the Everglades, introducing us to the flora and fauna of this watery wilderness.

Cerulean, Susan (ed.). *The Book of the Everglades.* Minneapolis, MN: Milkweed Editions, 2002. One volume in Milkweed's Literature for a Land Ethic series, this book is a collection of essays celebrating the Everglades while documenting the politics that threaten or support its restoration.

Douglas, Marjory Stoneman. *The Everglades: River of Grass.* Sarasota, FL: Pineapple Press, 2007. This classic, now in its 60th anniversary edition, begins with the words, "There are no other Everglades in the world" and traces the history of the people who have influenced the Glades for better or for worse.

Grunwald, Michael. *The Swamp: The Everglades, Florida, and the Politics of Paradise.* New York: Simon & Schuster, 2006. Divided into three parts, "The Natural Everglades," "Draining the Everglades," and "Restoring the Everglades," this book traces the area's historical and political trajectory over time.

Levin, Ted. *Liquid Land: A Journey through the Florida Everglades.* Athens, GA: University of Georgia Press, 2004. Levin takes us deep into the Everglades environment, telling the story of many of its inhabitants, from alligators to snail kites, and the human impact on it all.

SOCIAL HISTORY

Brown, Loren G. "Totch." *Totch: A Life in the Everglades.* Gainesville, FL: University Press of Florida, 1993. In this memoir, the author writes of his experiences in the Everglades City area as a young schoolboy; as a fisherman, crabber, and hunter; as a "pothauler"; as a decorated war veteran; and as a devoted husband, father, and grandfather.

McIver, Stuart B. *Death in the Everglades: The Murder of Guy Bradley, America's First Martyr to Environmentalism.* Gainesville, FL: University Press of Florida, 2009. Flamingo-area game warden Guy Bradley was murdered in 1905 while enforcing then-new Florida bird-protection laws. Author/documentary filmmaker McIver vividly recounts the story.

Perez, Larry. *Words on the Wilderness: A History of Place Names in South Florida's National Parks.* Everglades City, FL: ECity Publishing, 2007. National Park Service interpretive ranger Larry Perez has traced the origins of many of the place names in Everglades National Park as well as locations in Big Cypress National Preserve.

Simmons, Glen, and Laura Ogden. *Gladesmen: Gator Hunters, Moonshiners, and Skiffers.* Gainesville, FL: University Press of Florida, 1998. Simmons teams up with anthropologist Ogden to relate his experiences of fishing, gator hunting, and camping in the south Everglades, and to describe life in the little settlement called Flamingo.

Storter, Rob. *Crackers in the Glade: Life and Times in the Old Everglades.* Athens, GA: University of Georgia Press, 2000. With a foreword by Peter Matthiessen, and wonderfully illustrated with watercolors and pencil drawings by the author's own hand, Storter's memoir tells of early times in Everglades City. He writes of hundreds of pompano jumping into the air at a time; of 40,000 birds roosting on Duck Rock; and of the Chokoloskee postmaster selling groceries, delivering babies, and pulling teeth.

Tebeau, Charlton W. *Man in the Everglades: 2000 Years of Human History in the Everglades National Park.* Coral Gables, FL: University of Miami Press, 1968. Tebeau's short but thorough volume traces human habitation that includes the early Calusa; the Seminole and the years of "Indian removal"; the pioneers at Chatham Bend, Opossum Key, and the rivers to the south; and the settlements at Cape Sable and Flamingo.

Will, Lawrence E. *A Dredgeman of Cape Sable.* Belle Glade, FL: The Glades Historical Society, 1984. Especially if you intend to paddle the Bear Lake Canoe Trail, you will want to read the story of one of the men who dredged this waterway, battling the heat and mosquitoes and all the hardships that came with digging a channel through this mangrove wilderness.

POETRY AND FICTION

Magers, Rick. *Dark Caribbean.* Charleston, SC: BookSurge Publishing, 2007. Read this novel if you're curious about a time when many in the Everglades City area became involved in the drug trade. It's written by one who was involved. Magers says, "Changed my name . . . don't mind being hung for som'n I did, but I'll be damned if I'll hand 'em the rope."

Matthiessen, Peter. *Shadow Country*. New York: Modern Library, 2008. Called "a new rendering of the Watson legend," *Shadow Country* is a compilation of three of Matthiessen's novels (*Killing Mister Watson, Lost Man's River,* and *Bone by Bone*) that tell the story of Ed Watson and his 1910 death at Smallwood Store on Chokoloskee Island.

Mitchell, Roger. *The One Good Bite in the Saw-grass Plant.* New York: Natural Dam Publishing, 2010. This collection of poems is a celebration of the Everglades as experienced by the author during an artist's residency in the park.

Sullivan, Anne McCrary. *Ecology II: Throat Song from the Everglades.* Cincinnati, OH: WordTech Editions, 2009. Poetry and science merge in this collection of poems that traces an arc from grief to recovery through interaction with the plants and animals of Everglades National Park.

FIELD GUIDES

Alden, Peter, Rick Cech, and Gil Nelson. *National Audubon Society Field Guide to Florida.* New York: Alfred A. Knopf, 1998. This compact Audubon guide highlights some of the many plant and animal species found in Florida, describes the state's ecosystems and weather, and provides star charts.

Nellis, David W. *Seashore Plants of South Florida and the Caribbean: A Guide to Identification and Propagation of Xeriscape Plants.* Sarasota, FL: Pineapple Press, 1994. Excellent to carry along if you're going to beach sites, this guide will not only help you know what you're looking at, but also tell you about historical uses of these plants and the role each plant plays in the ecology of its location.

PADDLING GUIDES

Brighton, Patrick, MD. *Paddlers' Guide for Treating Medical Emergencies.* Birmingham, AL: Menasha Ridge Press, 2006. This small volume written by a physician with a sense of humor offers entertaining and sometimes downright hilarious reading, while providing serious information about what to do in medical emergencies on the water.

Johnson, Shelley. *Sea Kayaking: A Woman's Guide.* Camden, ME: Ragged Mountain Press, 1998. Well-illustrated and comprehensive, this guide explains gear, essential skills, and navigation strategies, and includes sections on "Paddling while Pregnant," "Paddling with the Family," and "To Pee or Not to Pee."

Molloy, Johnny. *A Paddler's Guide to Everglades National Park.* Gainesville, FL: University Press of Florida, 2009. Molloy's classic guidebook, now in its second edition, offers a comprehensive description of more than 60 paddling routes in and around Everglades National Park.

Ripple, Jeff. *Day Paddling Florida's 10,000 Islands and Big Cypress Swamp.* Woodstock, VT: Backcountry Guides, 2004. Ripple's guide focuses on paddles in the northern areas of Everglades National Park and in Big Cypress Swamp, and offers interesting and well-informed sidebars on flora and fauna.

APPENDIX 7: EVERGLADES WILDERNESS WATERWAY GPS COORDINATES

Flamingo: N25° 8.624' W80° 55.354'

U.S. Coast Guard (USCG) marker 1: N25° 11.033' W80° 54.748'

South Joe River Chickee: N25° 13.320' W81° 00.641'

Joe River Chickee: N25° 16.789' W81° 03.942'

Oyster Bay Chickee: N25° 19.410' W81° 03.981'

Wilderness Waterway (WW) marker 2: N25° 20.125' W81° 03.232'

WW marker 3: N25° 21.178' W81° 03.969'

Shark River Chickee: N25° 22.180' W81° 02.804'

WW marker 6: N25° 22.283' W81° 02.666'

WW marker 8: N25° 23.287' W81° 00.766'

Canepatch Campsite: N25° 25.317' W80° 56.619'

WW marker 9: N25° 24.903' W81° 00.441'

WW marker 11: N25° 25.851' W81° 04.856'

WW marker 12 & Harney River Chickee: N25° 25.953' W81° 05.464'

WW marker 14: N25° 26.597' W81° 05.983'

WW marker 16: N25° 27.027' W81° 05.567'

WW marker 17: N25° 26.955' W81° 08.173'

WW marker 19: N25° 27.096' W81° 08.427'

WW marker 21: N25° 27.097' W81° 08.538'

WW marker 23: N25° 27.347' W81° 08.971'

WW marker 24: N25° 28.458' W81° 08.659'

WW marker 25: N25° 28.611' W81° 08.737'

Broad River Campsite: N25° 28.748' W81° 08.534'

Highland Beach Campsite: N25° 28.677' W81° 11.079'

Camp Lonesome: N25° 29.292' W80° 59.994'

WW marker 26: N25° 30.097' W81° 02.434'

WW marker 28: N25° 31.120' W81° 02.260'

WW marker 29: N25° 31.527' W81° 02.495'

WW marker 31: N25° 31.850' W81° 02.810'

WW marker 32: N25° 32.386' W81° 02.899'

Rodgers River Chickee: N25° 32.138' W81° 03.742'

WW marker 34: N25° 32.710' W81° 02.940'

WW marker 35: N25° 33.018' W81° 03.061'

WW marker 36: N25° 33.222' W81° 03.078'

WW marker 37: N25° 33.972' W81° 04.074'

WW marker 38: N25° 34.013' W81° 04.174'

Willy Willy Campsite: N25° 34.840' W81° 03.333'

WW marker 42: N25° 33.989' W81° 05.709'

WW marker 44: N25° 34.114' W81° 05.968'

WW marker 45: N25° 34.294' W81° 06.017'

WW marker 46: N25° 34.293' W81° 06.988'

WW marker 47: N25° 34.554' W81° 07.412'

WW marker 49: N25° 34.561' W81° 07.438'

WW marker 50: N25° 34.611' W81° 07.736'

WW marker 51: N25° 34.749' W81° 08.088'

WW marker 52: N25° 34.924' W81° 08.331'

WW marker 53: N25° 35.502' W81° 08.337'

WW marker 55: N25° 36.060' W81° 08.403'

WW marker 56: N25° 36.554' W81° 08.049'

WW marker 58: N25° 36.904' W81° 07.924'

WW marker 59: N25° 37.325' W81° 08.510'

WW marker 60: N25° 38.040' W81° 08.550'

Lostmans Five Campsite: N25° 38.039' W81° 08.551'

WW marker 62: N25° 38.247' W81° 08.648'

WW marker 63: N25° 38.401' W81° 08.748'

Plate Creek Chickee: N25° 38.459' W81° 08.949'

WW marker 65: N25° 38.797' W81° 09.033'

WW marker 68: N25° 39.310' W81° 09.125'

WW marker 70: N25° 39.772' W81° 09.463'

WW marker 72: N25° 39.986' W81° 09.784'

WW marker 73: N25° 40.322' W81° 10.155'

WW marker 75: N25° 40.652' W81° 10.450'

WW marker 77: N25° 40.944' W81° 11.089'

WW marker 79: N25° 41.000' W81° 11.459'

WW marker 81: N25° 41.140' W81° 11.584'

WW marker 83: N25° 41.262' W81° 11.548'

WW marker 86: N25° 41.390' W81° 11.638'

Darwin's Place: N25° 41.650' W81° 12.133'

WW marker 87: N25° 41.674' W81° 12.162'

WW marker 88: N25° 41.796' W81° 12.196'

WW marker 89: N25° 42.010' W81° 12.320'

WW marker 91: N25° 42.086' W81° 12.457'

WW marker 93: N25° 42.696' W81° 12.471'

WW marker 95: N25° 42.939' W81° 12.777'

WW marker 97: N25° 43.218' W81° 12.934'

WW marker 99: N25° 43.291' W81° 13.415'

The Watson Place: N25° 42.551' W81° 14.737'

Sweetwater Chickee: N25° 44.617' W81° 12.685'

WW marker 107: N25° 44.844' W81° 14.987'

WW marker 108: N25° 45.261' W81° 15.377'

WW marker 109: N25° 45.347' W81° 15.487'

WW marker 110: N25° 45.646' W81° 15.559'

WW marker 112: N25° 45.823' W81° 15.646'

WW marker 113: N25° 46.342' W81° 15.928'

WW marker 114: N25° 46.543' W81° 15.937'

WW marker 115: N25° 46.685' W81° 16.143'

WW marker 116: N25° 46.801' W81° 16.089'

WW marker 117: N25° 46.837' W81° 16.190'

WW marker 119: N25° 46.915' W81° 16.386'

WW marker 120: N25° 47.084' W81° 16.456'

WW marker 121: N25° 47.422' W81° 16.602'

WW marker 123: N25° 48.050' W81° 17.363'

WW marker 125: N25° 48.123' W81° 17.589'

Crooked Creek Chickee: N25° 47.785' W81° 17.922'

WW marker 126: N25° 47.686' W81° 17.816'

Lopez River Campsite: N25° 47.275' W81° 18.374'

WW marker 127: N25° 47.320' W81° 20.201'

Chokoloskee Island: N25° 48.537' W81° 21.422'

Gulf Coast Visitor Center: N25° 50.730' W81° 23.234'

INDEX

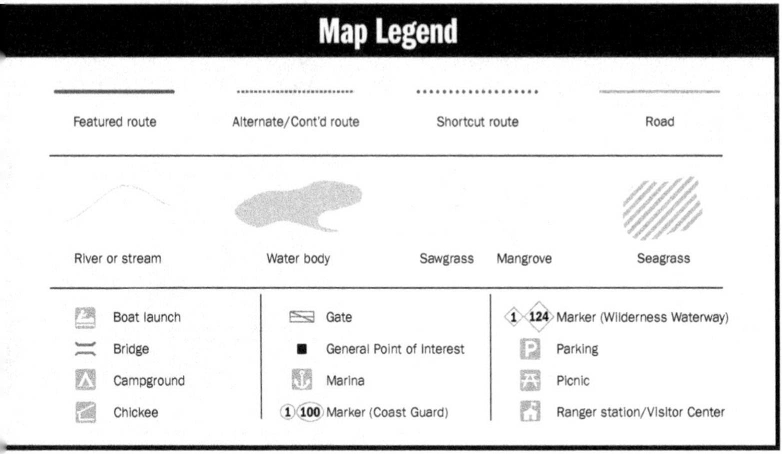
Map Legend
Featured route
Alternate/Cont'd route
Shortcut route
Road
River or stream
Water body
Sawgrass
Mangrove
Seagrass
Boat launch
Bridge
Campground
Chickee
Gate
General Point of Interest
Marina
1 100 Marker (Coast Guard)
1 124 Marker (Wilderness Waterway)
Parking
Picnic
Ranger station/Visitor Center

ABOUT THE AUTHORS

Authors **Holly Genzen** and **Anne McCrary Sullivan** began frequent paddling trips on the Everglades Wilderness Waterway 8 years ago. Both are Florida Master Naturalists certified by the University of Florida.

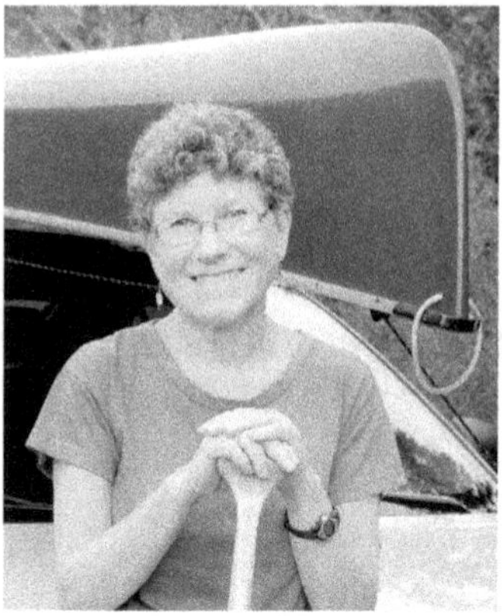

▶ A longtime outdoor adventurer, **Holly Genzen** has a master's degree in outdoor education and a PhD in educational administration; she was an associate professor at National Louis University. An avid hiker, she has solo thru-hiked the Appalachian Trail, and in recent years, she has focused her canoeing and kayaking activities on Florida's many springs, rivers, and coastal trails. She has been a volunteer resident at former President and Mrs. Hoover's Camp Rapidan in Shenandoah National Park, and she is a volunteer at Trout Lake Nature Center in Eustis, Florida. Holly lives in Leesburg, Florida, with her husband, Gary, and cat, Sherman.

▶ In a small wooden boat, with her marine biologist mother, **Anne McCrary Sullivan** had her earliest water adventures before she was old enough to walk. She is now an avid paddler and a naturalist volunteer in Everglades National Park. She first visited the park as an artist in residence, and her book of poems, *Ecology II: Throat Song from the Everglades* (WordTech Editions; Cincinnati, OH; 2009), explores flora, fauna, and ecology through a poetic lens. She has an MFA in poetry and a PhD in English education, and is recently retired from National Louis University where she was a professor of interdisciplinary studies.

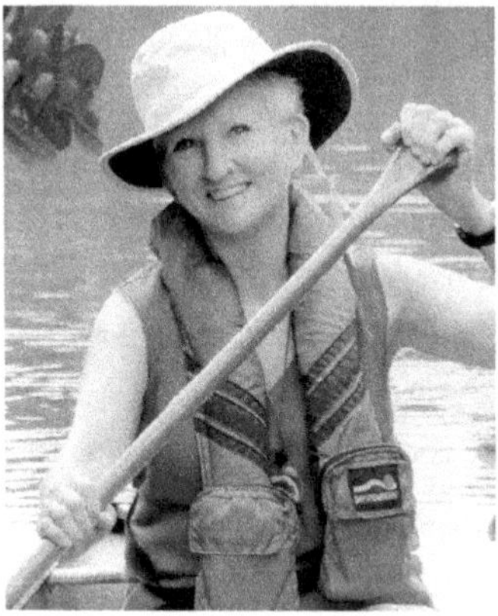

DEAR CUSTOMERS AND FRIENDS,

SUPPORTING YOUR INTEREST IN OUTDOOR ADVENTURE, travel, and an active lifestyle is central to our operations, from the authors we choose to the locations we detail to the way we design our books. Menasha Ridge Press was incorporated in 1982 by a group of veteran outdoorsmen and professional outfitters. For many years now, we've specialized in creating books that benefit the outdoors enthusiast.

Almost immediately, Menasha Ridge Press earned a reputation for revolutionizing outdoors- and travel-guidebook publishing. For such activities as canoeing, kayaking, hiking, backpacking, and mountain biking, we established new standards of quality that transformed the whole genre, resulting in outdoor-recreation guides of great sophistication and solid content. Menasha Ridge continues to be outdoor publishing's greatest innovator.

The folks at Menasha Ridge Press are as at home on a white-water river or mountain trail as they are editing a manuscript. The books we build for you are the best they can be, because we're responding to your needs. Plus, we use and depend on them ourselves.

We look forward to seeing you on the river or the trail. If you'd like to contact us directly, join in at www.trekalong.com or visit us at www.menasharidge.com. We thank you for your interest in our books and the natural world around us all.

SAFE TRAVELS,

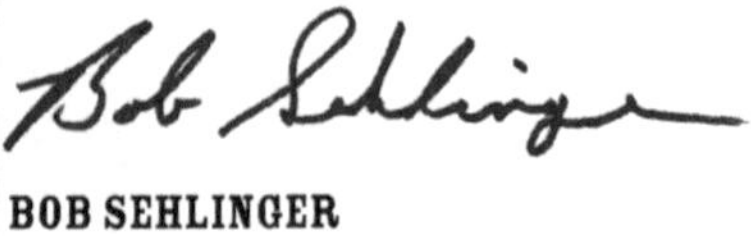

BOB SEHLINGER
PUBLISHER

Printed in the USA
CPSIA information can be obtained
at www.ICGtesting.com
JSHW011521130424
61126JS00002B/4

9 780897 328982